HULL COLLEGE

A bloke's
diagnose-it-yourself
guide to health

A bloke's diagnose-it-yourself guide to health

**Dr Keith Hopcroft
and Dr Alistair Moulds**

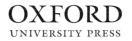

OXFORD
UNIVERSITY PRESS

OXFORD

UNIVERSITY PRESS

Great Clarendon Street, Oxford OX2 6DP, UK

Oxford New York

Athens Auckland Bangkok Bogota Buenos Aires Calcutta Cape Town Chennai Dar es Salaam Delhi Florence Hong Kong Istanbul Karachi Kuala Lumpur Madrid Melbourne Mexico City Mumbai Nairobi Paris São Paulo Singapore Taipei Tokyo Toronto Warsaw

and associated companies in
Berlin Ibadan

Oxford is a trade mark of Oxford University Press
Published in the United States by Oxford University Press, Inc., New York

© K. Hopcroft and A. Moulds, 2000

The moral rights of the author have been asserted

First published 2000

A catalogue record for this title is available from the
British Library

Library of Congress Cataloging in Publication Data
(Data available)

1 3 5 7 9 10 8 6 4 2

ISBN 0 19 262825 9
Typeset by J & L Composition Ltd, Filey, North Yorkshire
Printed in Great Britain on acid free paper by Biddles Ltd.,
Guildford & King's Lynn

Foreword

Blokes are famed for not taking their health as seriously as they should, but I suspect that this has more to do with ignorance than bravado – when something does go wrong men invariably need more support and nurturing than their better halves! But good reliable information on men's health is surprisingly hard to come by, and what little there is tends to concentrate on six packs and biceps, rather than hearts and testicles. *A Bloke's DIY Guide to Health* fills that gap perfectly, Keith and Alistair's easy to follow style and no-nonsense approach have resulted in a gem of a book – if only it was available on the NHS!

Mark Porter

Contents

Men behaving healthily?

Why another book on men's health? Because this one's different. Almost no preaching, a focus on quality rather than quantity of life, and a unique diagnose-it-yourself guide to every symptom a bloke is likely to suffer. And why should you buy it? It depends on whether you're a bloke, a bloke's partner, or a bloke's mum:

a bloke – buy it because you hate going to the doctor and it will probably mean you don't have to; or get it to impress your partner that, maybe, you're taking your health seriously at last;

a bloke's partner – buy it because he never sees the doc and this way you can bring the doc to him; or to show that you care; or to solve a birthday, Christmas, or Valentine's day present problem; or because he's been whining on about some symptom for ages but not done anything about it and you simply want to shut him up;

a bloke's mum – buy it because he doesn't look after himself properly and, hey, you're still his mum.

Now you've bought it, we're going to let you in on two major health secrets. Whenever doctors write about men's health, they make a very big deal about the fact that, compared to women, blokes up to the age of about 50 make less use of the health service – especially their GP. Various neat theories have been put forward to explain this, such as:

- women go to the doctor for services like family planning and cervical smears
- women get used to seeing the doctor for their kids and this makes them more likely to attend for themselves too
- men are 'risk takers' and so tend to ignore symptoms
- men are traditionally stoical
- men worry they might lose their jobs if they're absent because of illness or appointments with the doctor

- the health service doesn't cater properly for the working man
- men simply don't like seeing doctors,

and so on. But we think there may be another reason, and this is our first secret: *maybe men don't come to the doctor because they've got it right – they don't need to.*

The vast majority of symptoms – particularly in blokes aged 15–50 – are nothing much to worry about. They either go away on their own or they're irrelevant. Perhaps men have sussed this out and so make a conscious decision not to spend their time seeking reassurance from the doctor. Of course, just occasionally, they'll get it wrong, and that lump or pain they've been ignoring will unfortunately turn out to be something nasty.

On the other hand, it may be that all this doctor avoidance is just a macho front covering up the fact that blokes are plain scared of what their doctor might tell them. So maybe they just hope that most medical problems are insignificant, and get it right more by luck than judgement. In the meantime, they're putting up with the worry which comes with uncertainty.

If only there was an easy, DIY way of working out what symptoms mean, which can be safely ignored, which can be self-treated, and which should be taken to the GP or hospital. Well, now there is, and you're reading it. Because – and this is secret number two – *with just a little guidance, it's not difficult to sort out most of your symptoms.* Doctors know that 90% of the information needed to make a diagnosis

comes just from the 'history' – what you tell the doctor. Contrary to popular belief, examining a patient usually only helps the doc a little, and special tests even less. In fact, most physical check-overs are done either to confirm to the doctor what he already reckons is wrong, or to reassure the patient that his problem is being taken seriously. This is how doctors can diagnose pretty accurately many problems over the telephone.

Our diagnose-it-yourself guide exploits this fact by supplying *you* with the information you need to make easy, step-by-step self-diagnoses, and then giving you the low-down on what to do about your particular problem.

We're not going to pretend that the book will get it right 100% of the time. Illnesses don't read textbooks and so they'll sometimes show themselves in odd or unpredictable ways, and there's always the occasional rarity which can catch us all out – so the general rule is that, if you're in doubt, you should consult your GP. But, if you read the information carefully and sensibly, then, most of the time, this book will give you a pretty clear idea of what's going on and what to do about it.

Two final points: we're aware that doctors can be female as well as male. We use the male form throughout to avoid clumsy sentences and political correctness – and because blokes usually see male GPs. We're also aware that a proportion of males are homosexuals. Most of the book is written with the heterosexual in mind, but we do highlight the occasional area where a symptom might be of special importance to homosexuals.

Keith Hopcroft
Alistair Moulds
October 1999

How to use this book

Part One, *'How to get a good seeing to'*, gives tips on getting medical help when you need it and making the most of seeing your GP. Part Three, *'Live fast and die old'*, looks at lifestyle and how it affects health. We've deliberately avoided a preachy approach in this particular section because: (a) we think life is about quality as much as quantity; (b) some traditionally 'frowned-upon' activities aren't half as bad as originally thought and may even be good for you; and (c) we don't want you to bin the book.

Sandwiched between these sections is the Part Two, *'diagnose-it-yourself'* guide: virtually all the common symptoms you're likely to suffer are included. So here's how you become your own doctor.

Step one: *check your age*. This book is aimed at 'blokes', who we arbitrarily define as men in the 15–50 age bracket. The older you are – and particularly if you're above 50 – the greater the likelihood that a symptom you're suffering might have a significant cause. So although those of you over 50 might find the flow charts useful and interesting, you should *not* rely on them, and you should have a lower threshold for seeing your GP.

Step two: *find your symptom*. The symptoms are arranged in alphabetical order. If a quick flick through the contents draws a blank, use the index to find the page you need.

Step three: *follow the chart*. A series of simple yes/no questions should lead you to the diagnosis. Each diagnosis has extra clues to help you check you've got it right. Every so often, you might come across these logos: ⚠ and ⚠. The first means you'll need to see your GP sharpish, the second that you need urgent medical help. They're on the charts to get important information across quickly and clearly, and to make the pages prettier.

Step four: *find out how likely your diagnosis is and what it means*. The information accompanying the flow chart gives more detail about your problem and explains what you should do about it. Note: if you've ended up with a 'Only rare causes left' diagnosis then either you've got an unusual problem or you've got it wrong. It's worth thinking again and trying another run through the flow chart.

That's it. Bloke, heal thyself.

Part One

How to get a good seeing to

Seeing the doc can be a stressful business. Apart from the obvious worry about what he might say or do, simply trying to sort out an appointment can make you uptight. So it's worth remembering that there are some alternatives.

Your local chemist: if you think you need something for a minor problem like a cough, cold, or tummy bug, this should be your first stop. But your chemist sells more than just cough linctuses, vitamins, anti-diarrhoea treatments, and the like. Some very effective treatments which, until fairly recently, you could only get on prescription have become available over the counter. Examples include ibuprofen (an anti-inflammatory drug for pains and strains), hydrocortisone 1% cream (for eczema), and cimetidine (a powerful antacid). The pharmacist can help you choose the right treatment for your problem, and he'll direct you to your GP if he thinks that's who you really need to see.

Casualty: how do you know if you're right to have pitched up in casualty? Simple: remember it's also known as the 'accident and emergency department'. So just ask yourself, 'Am I an accident or an emergency?' If the answer is yes, you're in the right place. If not, then go quickly and quietly before you embarrass yourself. The information box below should help if you're not sure.

Sexually transmitted disease clinics: these are mentioned at various points in the book, and have lots of other names (like 'clap clinic', 'department of genitourinary medicine', and 'special clinic'). They specialize in patients who have picked up germs passed on through sex – most local hospitals have a clinic of this sort. And how can you tell if you might have a sexually transmitted disease? You might have a severe burning pain when you pee, and a discharge from your penis, or both; or your penis might develop an ulcer (or ulcers). For more information, see the 'Penis sores

Problems which should be taken to casualty

NB This is for guidance only - and there's nothing to stop you taking a quick look at the appropriate flow chart in this book if you're in doubt.

- significant injury to limbs or trunk (e.g. possible broken bone, a cut which might need stitching)
- head injury (if a severe bump, knocked out for any length of time, loss of memory, or drowsiness)
- an eye injury
- a knee injury with sudden swelling (i.e. within minutes)
- all but the mildest burns
- severe chest pain
- severe shortness of breath
- severe, constant pain in the abdomen
- sudden, severe headache with drowsiness and/or vomiting
- vomiting blood (except a few streaks after a lot of retching)
- any overdose (deliberate or accidental)
- poisoning
- any loss of consciousness (other than a faint, or a fit if you're known to be epileptic and you recover from it quickly)
- sudden, severe pain in the testicle
- inability to pass urine (at all)
- feeling depressed to the point of suicide

and/or discharge' section. All you have to do is phone your local hospital, ask for the special clinic, and find out when to go along (usually within a day or two). Of course, you could see your GP instead, but he's likely to point you in the direction of the clinic anyway, because you'll probably need some special tests – and they'll probably want to check out your partner too.

The receptionist at your doctor's surgery: in these days of staff training, corporate image, and customer satisfaction, you're more likely to be greeted by a cheesy grin and a 'How may I help you?' than be lightly toasted by the archetypal fire-breathing dragon. Probably. Whatever, bear in mind that the receptionist is likely to have access to loads of medical information and services. A brief mention of your problem may result, for example, in you being given a health education leaflet, sent to the practice nurse (e.g. to

have some stitches taken out or for travel vaccinations), or pointed in the direction of a local self-help group. The receptionist can also give you a practice leaflet – every practice has one – outlining the staff, facilities, and opening times of your surgery.

The telephone: telephone advice lines for health problems are becoming very popular. Some are local while others are being developed nationally, such as NHS Direct **NHS Direct 0845 4647** which provides information on health problems and NHS services. You can pretty much guarantee that, whatever your problem, someone, somewhere, is on the end of a phone line waiting for your call. As a starting point, try the phone book, directory enquiries, or NHS Direct. Remember, too, that doctors can often save you the hassle of booking an appointment by dealing with many problems over the telephone – including some requests for certificates and prescriptions, and many illnesses (if you don't believe us, try reading the book's introductory blurb again). Your doctor may have a specific slot for telephone consultations – check the practice leaflet. Alternatively, phone his receptionist to leave him a message.

This book: the flow charts and the explanatory blurb will tell you when and how to self-treat and when you really need to see an expert.

So there are lots of sources of medical help available. But what if you've decided that it's time to bite the bullet and see your GP? How can you get to see him with the minimum amount of hassle? And, once you're there, how do you make the most of it?

How to see your GP

Shouting, 'Let me through, I'm a patient' is unlikely to work. You'll have more success if you know a bit about the 'system'. These days, most GPs run an appointment system – simply phone up and book a consultation. Avoid Monday mornings if you can, as this is usually melt-down time for the surgery switchboard. When it's hectic and difficult to get through, you're probably better off pitching up at the surgery and speaking to a receptionist.

Receptionists have a tough job. On the one hand, they're trying to satisfy the queue of customers and on the other they're responsible for keeping the doctors' surgeries running smoothly, without unnecessary interruptions. And, in the meantime, they have to answer the phone, deal with queries, file records, and so on. So if you're asked a few questions, bear in mind that they're only trying to get enough information to deal with your request properly. If you feel embarrassed talking within earshot of other people, just explain that you'd rather discuss matters somewhere private.

Whether you've phoned up or turned up, how quickly you'll be seen depends on how busy the practice is at the time and how urgent your problem is. If you feel that it really can't wait for the next 'routine' slot that you're offered, then say so: any system should be flexible enough to allow for the occasional 'urgent' case. And if you still feel that your problem isn't being taken seriously, point this out – politely and assertively, but not aggressively. Maybe the receptionist hasn't heard you properly, doesn't understand that you have what you think might be an urgent problem, or doesn't realize how worried you are: tell her. Genuinely alarming symptoms like chest pain or shortness of breath, when explained to the receptionist, usually prompt pretty rapid action.

If your GP works in a group practice (in other words, with a team of other doctors, as most do), one useful tip is to say that you're not really bothered which doctor you see. One of the other docs in the practice may be less booked up than your usual GP so you might be able to get a more convenient appointment. This is fine for one-off problems – but if you're consulting about a long-term medical complaint which your GP has been dealing with, it's better to stick with your usual doc, as he'll know all the background.

Some surgeries run an 'open access' service where patients can just turn up and be seen on a 'first come, first served' basis. This saves messing around negotiating appointment times with receptionists, but can lead to mind-numbingly long waits, so take a good book or check out the quietest times.

You might be lucky and discover that your doctor is very consumer-friendly and so runs late evening ('commuter') or Saturday morning surgeries to provide slots for punters who are at work during normal opening hours. To find out what sort of service your GP provides and how the system works, speak to a friendly receptionist or take a look at the practice leaflet.

If you're generally unhappy with the service your doctor provides, you've always got the option of looking for another practice. Ask around friends or neighbours for recommendations, or get some information from NHS Direct (0845 4647), or from the local Health Authority or Community Health Council (the phone numbers should be in the local directory). Or you could consider 'going private'. There aren't many private GPs about, although private 'walk-in' clinics are becoming increasingly popular, especially in large cities. Bear in mind, though, that any private doctor you see won't have the benefit of all your medical records and will probably not be able to provide the continuity of an NHS GP – and, whatever your problem, the bill you get is likely to make you feel even more ill.

Some private health organizations are very keen on pushing 'Well Man Checks'. These health MOTs sound great in theory but are probably virtually worthless. The tests they perform are hard to make sense of in someone who's 'well', and simply being given the all-clear on a medical is no insurance against illness, as anyone whose car has broken down the day after a service will confirm. And is it really worth forking out your hard-earned dosh just to have some smart doctor in plush consulting rooms telling you what you already know (that, say, you're a lard-arse who smokes and drinks too much, although he's likely to put it rather more politely)?

How to make the most of seeing your GP

The average GP has about nine minutes per consultation and sees around 18 patients in each surgery. Two surgeries a day are fitted in around home visits, paperwork, meetings teaching, and so on. So if your GP seems pressured, that's because he is. This isn't your problem, of course, but appreciating this will at least help you understand why he may have a brisk approach. Getting your symptoms, worries, and points of view over in a short time can be a tall order, especially if you're feeling a bit tense – as most people are when they visit the doctor. A bit of forward thinking and an understanding of what is likely to happen will help you get the most out of your visit to the doc. Your consultation will probably follow a standard pattern:

1. *he'll take a 'history'* – this simply means he'll ask you all about your problem, so try to get your facts straight before you see him. This will make the process feel more efficient and less like an interrogation. For example, if you have a pain, work out when it started, how often it happens, what it feels like, whether you've had it before, what makes it better or worse, and so on, because these are the things he's likely to ask you;

2. *he may want to examine you* (or at least the relevant 'bit') – so be prepared for this and don't be bashful;

3. *he might want to arrange some tests* – these might include blood tests and X-rays, although they're not necessary in most cases. If your problem has anything to do with your waterworks, take a specimen of your wee with you – the doc can do an easy 'dipstick' test on it there and then;

4. *he'll 'manage' your problem* – this might involve just reassurance and explanation, further tests, advice on self-help, a prescription, or the suggestion that you see a hospital specialist.

What if, by the end of the consultation, the doc hasn't dealt with a particular worry you had? Or maybe he doesn't seem to have taken your problem seriously? Or he hasn't given you a prescription or blood test when you thought

Things not to say to your GP

- 'I don't come very often so I've brought a list.'
- 'I just want some antibiotics.'
- 'I think I've got ME.'
- 'I've got toothache.'
- 'I need an X-ray.'
- 'I've got chronic pain in my solar plexus.'
- 'I just want a letter to see a specialist.'
- 'The TV/radio doc said . . .'/'I cut this out of a newspaper/magazine . . .'
- 'While I'm here, doctor . . .'

you needed one? If, for some reason, you're not totally satisfied, then tell him. The trick is, again, to be assertive without being aggressive – make it clear that you're not 100% happy and why, then give your GP a chance to explain his management of your problem again and discuss the situation further. Obviously, what a patient wants and what he actually needs aren't always the same thing – if this seems to be the sticking point, your doc will try to sort it out to your mutual satisfaction.

Apparently innocuous phrases patients sometimes use can grate with the average GP – perhaps because they can come across as a 'demand', or because he's heard the same thing hundreds of times in the past. We've highlighted and explained some examples – not to slate patients but to illustrate how an innocent remark runs the risk of messing up your consultation. Remember, you want the doc to be on your side. Knowing why these phrases might wind him up also gives you an insight into how his mind works and how he likes to do his job.

So what's wrong with the phrases in the box?

'*I don't come very often so I've bought a list.*' You may think you're being extra thoughtful by not bothering the doc too often and bringing the occasional 'job lot' instead. Your GP won't see it this way – he'll be wondering how he's going to get through your shopping list in nine minutes. The answer is simply not to bring lists. Instead, either spread the load over a couple of consultations if you really do have a lot of problems to get through, prioritize by letting your GP concentrate on the areas bothering you most, or just admit that your real problem is anxiety, which is why you've suddenly developed the habit of writing down lists of symptoms.

'*I just want some antibiotics.*' Your GP dislikes this gambit because: (a) the average punter is not always good at judging when antibiotics are really necessary; and (b) he'll antic-

ipate a battle. It's better to admit that the doc's years at medical school must count for something and let him make up his own mind what is the best treatment for your particular problem. You're perfectly entitled to ask if antibiotics might help, of course – at least you'll get an explanation, if not a prescription.

'*I think I've got ME.*' Guaranteed to send a shiver down his spine. Of course, you might be right (especially if you've read the 'Tired all the time' section), but the path to self-diagnosis (without this book) – particularly in controversial areas like ME – is littered with banana skins. The problem for the doc is, again, that he might feel you're undermining his professional opinion. It's better to let him make his own diagnosis then, if you're not convinced, ask him to explain why he doesn't think it's ME, or whatever you're concerned it might be.

'*I've got toothache.*' GPs are not dentists. Dentists are dentists. Dentists are trained to deal with dental problems and doctors are trained to deal with everything but. GPs get tetchy having to deal with toothache simply because they're cheaper (i.e. free) or more accessible than the dentist. Solution: see a dentist.

'*I want an X-ray.*' Same problem as for antibiotics (above).

'*I've got chronic pain in my solar plexus.*' The problem with this type of opener is the use of medical language – patients sometimes use medical words and phrases inaccurately. At best, this can cause amusement (as in, 'My hydrofoil's getting bigger, doc' – see hydrocele) and, at worst, dangerous confusion. Chronic pain, in doctorspeak, means pain going on a long time, not pain that is severe. And God knows what or where the solar plexus really is. We don't. It's best to stick to simple language and avoid technical terms unless you're sure you've got them right.

'*I just want a note for a specialist.*' This belittles one of the GP's key roles: that of 'gatekeeper' to specialist services. GPs are trained to filter out those patients whose problems need dealing with at the hospital. They become very skilled at this and manage to sort out 90% of problems themselves. This doesn't mean that patients are being denied the care they need. It does mean that they're protected from unnecessary tests or unpleasant or harmful treatments, that waiting lists are kept to a reasonable level, and that the NHS remains more or less affordable. Again, if you really think your problem might need the services of a specialist then, once your doc has given his opinion, say so. That way you can both discuss the situation further and negotiate a way forward.

'*The TV/radio doc said . . .*'/'*I cut this out of a newspaper/magazine.*' The media's aim is to encourage people to watch more TV or buy more magazines or newspapers – not to provide a balanced account of medical news. All sense of perspective can be lost so the public's levels of anxiety and expectations are raised while the GP's molars are ground down. The most constructive approach is to ask for his views of something you've picked up from the media rather than automatically treat what the media doc said as gospel.

'*While I'm here, doctor* . . .' This scenario is also fondly known as the 'hand on knob' consultation. Here's how it works: punter attends with a trivial problem such as a cold; allocated nine minutes is spent discussing snot; punter is just about to leave when he reveals the real reason for coming (usually something he regards as embarrassing, like impotence). The insignificant problem (the cold) is known in the trade as a 'passport symptom', because it simply gets the patient into the consultation. The 'real' symptom is only revealed as he's leaving – hence 'hand on knob' – because he's actually used the consultation to judge whether the doc is sympathetic and to pluck up the courage to spill the beans. Problem? The doc has to start all over again on a time-consuming problem and is now running late. The solution is to try to be up front with your real problem from the outset. Whatever it is, you can guarantee your GP will have heard it all before.

We're aware, of course, that GPs also have annoying habits, such as when they put everything down to a virus (it often is), use complex medical terms (in an attempt to say something more impressive than 'It's a virus'), or ask patients apparently stupid questions like, 'What do *you* think might be wrong?' (usually asked because the patient's worries about possible causes are important, not because the doc is buggered if he knows what's wrong).

So the consultation's winding up, you've given your GP the information he needed, you've avoided any of the forbidden phrases, you've asked for clarification of his advice, but you're still not happy. What should you do? It's best to tell him, so you can make a sensible plan of what to do next. You'll notice that the key message from the 'irritating phrases' outlined above is that, while you should let your GP make his own mind up about your symptoms, it's always best to make sure you voice your concerns about your problem or how he's handled it. He would much rather you did this than leave the consultation totally dissatisfied. Maybe he's just having an off-day and your best bet is to cut your losses and come back another time. Or you've both taken it as far as you can but still can't see eye to eye – in which case, it's worth asking if you could have a second opinion (maybe from another doctor in the practice or from a specialist). And if all else fails, of course, at least you've got this book to refer to.

Part Two

Diagnose-it-yourself guide

Our flow charts are designed to lead you quickly and painlessly to the most likely diagnosis and, in the vast majority of
cases, will do just that. However, diseases cannot always be
relied upon to follow the usual pattern and may affect you in
a different or more worrying way to normal.

Make sure you read the 'How to use this book' section
before using the diagnose-it-yourself guide. And remember –
the flow charts are an aid. They are not a substitute for your
own common sense and judgement. If you have any doubts,
particularly when you're in a or ⚠ diagnosis area – if
your symptoms don't seem to fit a diagnosis or if they seem
worse or more serious than the chart suggests – then seek
medical advice.

Remember:

⚠ means see your GP sharpish

⚠ means an urgent hospital job

Abdominal pain – one-off

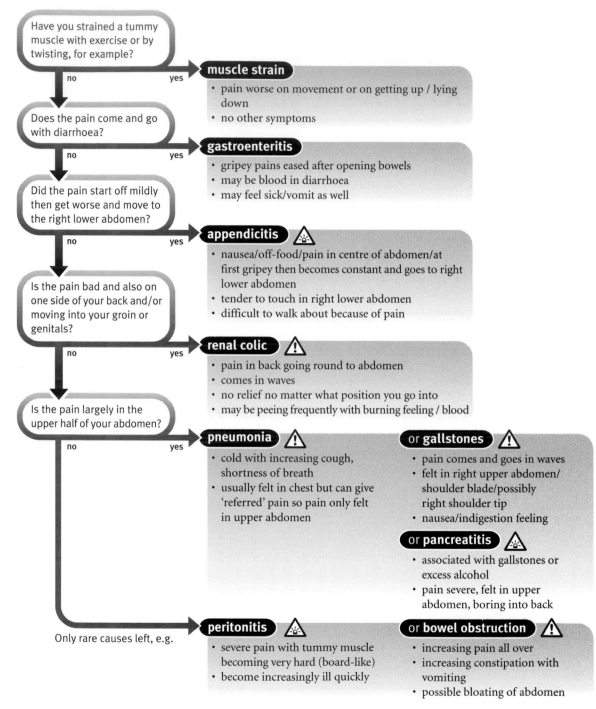

Have you strained a tummy muscle with exercise or by twisting, for example?

no   yes

muscle strain
- pain worse on movement or on getting up / lying down
- no other symptoms

Does the pain come and go with diarrhoea?

no   yes

gastroenteritis
- gripey pains eased after opening bowels
- may be blood in diarrhoea
- may feel sick/vomit as well

Did the pain start off mildly then get worse and move to the right lower abdomen?

no   yes

appendicitis
- nausea/off-food/pain in centre of abdomen/at first gripey then becomes constant and goes to right lower abdomen
- tender to touch in right lower abdomen
- difficult to walk about because of pain

Is the pain bad and also on one side of your back and/or moving into your groin or genitals?

no   yes

renal colic
- pain in back going round to abdomen
- comes in waves
- no relief no matter what position you go into
- may be peeing frequently with burning feeling / blood

Is the pain largely in the upper half of your abdomen?

no   yes

pneumonia
- cold with increasing cough, shortness of breath
- usually felt in chest but can give 'referred' pain so pain only felt in upper abdomen

or gallstones
- pain comes and goes in waves
- felt in right upper abdomen/ shoulder blade/possibly right shoulder tip
- nausea/indigestion feeling

or pancreatitis
- associated with gallstones or excess alcohol
- pain severe, felt in upper abdomen, boring into back

Only rare causes left, e.g.

peritonitis
- severe pain with tummy muscle becoming very hard (board-like)
- become increasingly ill quickly

or bowel obstruction
- increasing pain all over
- increasing constipation with vomiting
- possible bloating of abdomen

If your abdominal pain is severe, or you feel ill or faint with it, then the actual diagnosis does not matter – it is likely to have a serious cause and you must seek medical attention immediately.

Gastroenteritis A germ in the bowel, usually through something you've eaten – hence the term, 'food poisoning'.

Treatment The problem will sort itself out without any treatment, but it can take anything from a few hours to 10 days. All you need to do is drink plenty of clear fluids then start a light diet once any vomiting stops (the diarrhoea usually takes longer). If the trots are terrible, you may be tempted to get some medicine from the chemist to bung you up, but it's probably better to let the germ simply pass through the system. A hot water bottle and some paracetamol will help ease the gripey pain. Contact your GP if the diarrhoea's showing no signs of settling after 10 days, you're passing a lot of blood, or you've just travelled somewhere exotic. And if your job involves handling food, don't return to work until the diarrhoea has stopped for 48 hours, and be very careful about hand washing.

Muscle strain A pulled muscle in your abdomen can cause a mild pain.

Treatment Simple – use a painkiller and some heat, take it easy on the sports for a week or two, remember to warm up in future, and it should heal quickly.

Appendicitis The appendix is a useless, worm-like bit of gut. If it becomes inflamed, it swells and causes severe belly ache.

Treatment A hospital job to have it whipped out.

Renal colic This is a stone (usually like a small piece of gravel) in the tube joining the kidney to the bladder. This tube is very thin and muscular, and squeezes hard to push the stone through, causing horrendous pain. Some people have a tendency to keep making stones, and so can get repeated attacks.

Treatment It probably depends who it's quickest to get to – the local hospital or your GP. You'll be in so much pain you won't really care who sees you, you'll just want it sorted out asap. It needs strong painkillers, usually by injection, and a high fluid intake. If your GP does treat you, he may need to send you to hospital anyway if it doesn't quickly set-tle down and, especially if it's your first attack, you're likely to need further tests.

Gallstones Stones in the gall bladder, another useless part of the anatomy – a small bag that sits just under the liver. No one knows what causes them, but they can run in families, and they can give repeated attacks of severe belly ache.

Treatment During an attack of pain (technically, 'biliary colic') you'll need either strong painkillers from your GP or a trip to the hospital. If attacks are frequent and a real nuisance, then the only cure is an operation to remove the gall bladder – and a low fat diet while you're waiting.

Pneumonia This is a severe infection of the lungs. It inflames the lung lining (the pleura), leading to 'pleurisy'. This can cause referred pain in the belly (pain arising in one place – in this case, the lungs – but felt somewhere else).

Treatment See your GP asap as this needs antibiotics. It can make you quite ill, in which case you'll be sent to hospital.

Pancreatitis and peritonitis Inflammation of the pancreas and the lining of the guts, respectively. Pancreatitis can be caused by a virus, too much alcohol, and gallstones, amongst other things. Peritonitis is usually caused by a hole (a 'perforation') appearing in the bowel courtesy of, for example, appendicitis or a duodenal ulcer.

Treatment Urgent hospital attention needed for both.

Bowel obstruction If your gut gets blocked, the muscular walls of your bowel will squeeze to try to push past it. This causes, amongst other symptoms, severe belly ache. Although it's pretty rare, there are lots of different reasons why your bowel might get blocked – the commonest is probably 'adhesions' (gluey bits which can stick bits of bowel together after previous surgery – such as for appendicitis).

Treatment Your GP will send you to hospital if he thinks you have bowel obstruction.

Abdominal pain – recurrent

Is the pain you are getting pretty much exactly the same as you have had in the past?

yes / **no**

'abdominal pain–one off' see p.12

Is your pain gripey with bloating and wind, and worse when you are stressed?

no / **yes**

irritable bowel syndrome

- may be diarrhoea, often first thing in the morning
- mucus (slime) but *no* blood in diarrhoea
- in some people can give constipation rather than diarrhoea (in which case bowel motions are pellet-like – 'rabbit droppings') or even alternating episodes of both
- may keep coming back

Is your pain associated with a lot of indigestion / heartburn?

no / **yes**

gastritis/ulcer

- pain in pit of stomach
- may be relieved by food / antacids
- may wake you at 1–2 a.m.

or gallstones ⚠

- bouts of pain / comes and goes in waves
- felt in right upper abdomen/ shoulder blade/possibly right shoulder tip
- nausea/off food/perhaps worse after fatty meals

Is the pain bad and also on one side of your back and/or moving into your groin or genitals?

no / **yes**

renal colic ⚠

- may have increased peeing, burning, blood in pee
- pain may come for only a day or two at a time, but when present is severe
- comes in waves, no relief no matter what position you try

Is the pain largely in the upper half of your abdomen?

no / **yes**

pancreatitis ⚠

- associated with gallstones/excess alcohol
- pain severe – felt in upper abdomen, boring into back

or gallstones

see above

Do you really only get the pain when you are constipated?

no / **yes**

constipation

- crampy pains in left lower abdomen
- feels worse before you try to go to the toilet
- relieved once bowels move

Only rare causes left, e.g.

inflammatory bowel disease

- blood may be a prominent symptom
- get diarrhoea during the night
- may lose weight

or cancer of the bowel ⚠

- may be diarrhoea and/or constipation with blood
- may be losing weight
- may have feeling bowel doesn't empty properly

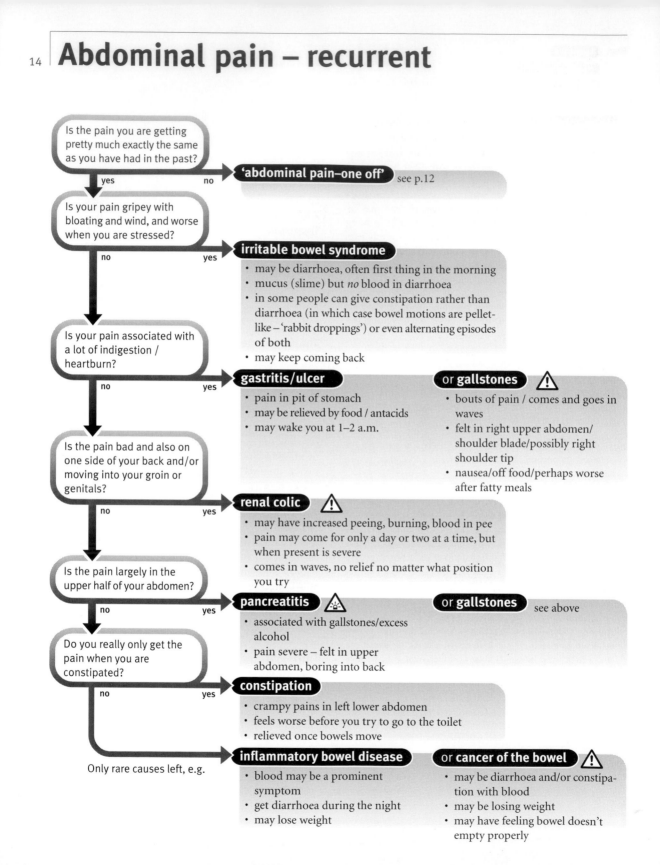

Irritable bowel syndrome (IBS)
The bowel is simply a long muscular tube. When 'irritable', it squeezes too much, too little, or in an uncoordinated way, resulting in the typical symptoms of IBS.

Treatment No one's absolutely sure what causes this problem – but it's very common, affecting up to one in five men, and, though troublesome, is harmless. Avoid any particular foods which you find aggravate it, increase your fibre if you get a lot of constipation, but decrease it if bloating is a big problem. It's worth cutting down on cigarettes, alcohol, and caffeine (in coffee, tea, and cola) too. Physical exercise, and relaxation exercises to reduce stress, may help. If the pain is very distressing then antispasmodic treatment, available from the chemist, may give some relief. And if it's getting really bad, or it's getting you down, discuss the problem with your GP, who may try other treatments – but bear in mind that there's no magic answer.

Gastritis/ulcer
The stomach produces acid to help digest the food. But sometimes the acid can inflame the stomach lining – 'gastritis' – causing an indigestion-type pain. Occasionally, the acid burns a small crater in the lining of the duodenum, the tube which carries food away from the stomach – this is a duodenal ulcer. This type of problem sometimes runs in families and can be caused, or aggravated, by alcohol, acidic medication (such as aspirin or ibuprofen), and a poor diet. A gastric ulcer is the same thing, but in the stomach – and it usually occurs in an older age group (the over 40s, whereas a duodenal ulcer affects blokes between the ages of 20 and 50).

Treatment For mild acid problems, look at your diet and lifestyle. Avoid spicy foods, eat regularly, and cut down on cigarettes and alcohol. Also, steer clear of some acidic over-the-counter painkillers like aspirin and ibuprofen; paracetamol is OK. The chemist will be able to give you an antacid which should sort you out. If the problem doesn't settle, or your symptoms point to an ulcer, see your GP – he can prescribe pretty powerful stuff to cut down the acid, and in some cases, treatments which might cure the problem once and for all.

Renal colic
This is explained in the 'Abdominal pain – one off' section. Some people tend to keep developing stones and so can suffer repeated attacks of renal colic.

Treatment The treatment of an attack is discussed in the 'Abdominal pain – one-off' section. If you get repeated attacks, your GP will have you checked out to see if there's any reason why you keep developing stones. It's important to drink plenty, and you may be given dietary advice, or some medication, to cut down the chances of further problems.

Constipation
If the bowel gets overloaded because you're not opening your bowels regularly, you are likely to feel vaguely uncomfortable most of the time – and suffer bouts of colicky pains as the bowel tries to squeeze stuff through.

Treatment Increase your fibre (such as fruit, veg, unprocessed bran) and fluid intake. Physical exercise helps too. Some medicines – especially painkillers – can cause constipation, so if you take something regularly, check with the chemist to see if it's the culprit. And while you're there, if all else has failed, think about using one of the multitude of over-the-counter laxatives – though just for a few days – to kick-start your bowel.

Gallstones
This is explained in the 'Abdominal pain – one-off' section. The pain may come back again, especially after fatty meals, until the problem is sorted out once and for all.

Treatment See the 'Abdominal pain – one-off' section. If attacks are frequent and a real nuisance, then the only cure is an operation to remove the gall bladder.

Pancreatitis
This is an inflamed pancreas – a bit of your innards which sits deep in the pit of your stomach and helps digest your food. It usually gets inflamed either because of gallstones or too much booze.

Treatment You shouldn't be in much doubt about what to do during an attack – the pain is bad and you'll feel pretty ill, so hospital is the obvious option. Preventing repeated attacks depends on the cause and might involve you having your gallstones sorted out or cutting out the booze.

Other medical problems
Very occasionally, repeated attacks of belly ache are caused by some other problem, such as a swollen kidney, inflammatory bowel disease (see p. 47), side-effects of medication, or bowel cancer (rare in the under 50s).

Treatment See your GP if you think you might have a problem of this sort – he will arrange any necessary tests.

Abnormal bowel motions

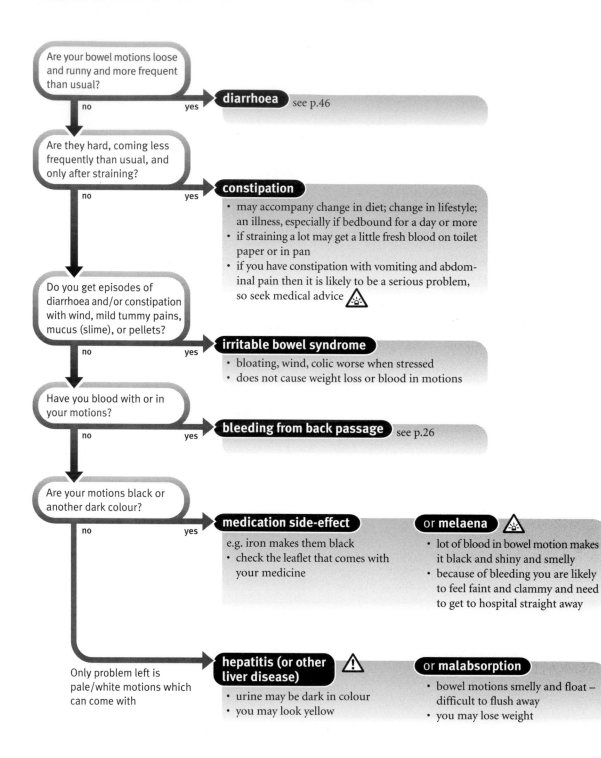

Are your bowel motions loose and runny and more frequent than usual?

no — yes →

diarrhoea see p.46

Are they hard, coming less frequently than usual, and only after straining?

no — yes →

constipation
- may accompany change in diet; change in lifestyle; an illness, especially if bedbound for a day or more
- if straining a lot may get a little fresh blood on toilet paper or in pan
- if you have constipation with vomiting and abdominal pain then it is likely to be a serious problem, so seek medical advice

Do you get episodes of diarrhoea and/or constipation with wind, mild tummy pains, mucus (slime), or pellets?

no — yes →

irritable bowel syndrome
- bloating, wind, colic worse when stressed
- does not cause weight loss or blood in motions

Have you blood with or in your motions?

no — yes →

bleeding from back passage see p.26

Are your motions black or another dark colour?

no — yes →

medication side-effect
e.g. iron makes them black
- check the leaflet that comes with your medicine

or melaena
- lot of blood in bowel motion makes it black and shiny and smelly
- because of bleeding you are likely to feel faint and clammy and need to get to hospital straight away

Only problem left is pale/white motions which can come with

hepatitis (or other liver disease)
- urine may be dark in colour
- you may look yellow

or malabsorption
- bowel motions smelly and float – difficult to flush away
- you may lose weight

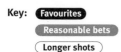
Diarrhoea See the 'Diarrhoea' section, p. 47.

Constipation This means difficulty in opening your bowels – in other words, having to strain a lot when you go. A hectic lifestyle, a poor diet, and a lack of exercise are the usual causes. Some medications (such as antidepressants and painkillers containing codeine) can bung you up – as can some illicit drugs (like heroin). A vicious cycle can develop: constipation might cause an anal fissure (see the 'Pain in the bottom' section) which, in turn, makes you unwilling to go, causing further constipation. Rarely, constipation coming on suddenly over a day or two can be the result of a blockage in your bowel ('intestinal obstruction'). This can be caused by a number of things and also results in severe belly ache and swelling, and vomiting.

Treatment Increase your fibre intake. This means more fruit, vegetables, and bran. Also, take more exercise, as this helps stimulate the bowels. Try to make use of the early morning urge to go, which usually comes on about half an hour after eating breakfast – so give yourself an extra 10 minutes in the morning to sit on the loo. If you think that some medication you're taking may be causing the problem, have a word with your chemist or GP, as you may be able to stop it or try an alternative. And while you're in the chemist's, you might try a laxative, such as senna tablets: this will help get you going, though it's best used only for a short time while you're sorting out your diet and some exercise. If you get a real pain in the bottom when you try to go, you've probably got an anal fissure – see the 'Pain in the bottom' section (p. 98) for advice on how to treat this. Constipation caused by intestinal obstruction needs urgent medical treatment – go to casualty.

Irritable bowel syndrome See the 'Diarrhoea' (p. 47) and 'Abdominal pain – recurrent' (p. 14) sections for details about this condition and how it's treated. If you suffer from irritable bowel syndrome, you can get constipation or diarrhoea, or both – and you may pass mucus and stuff that looks like rabbit droppings.

Bleeding from back passage See the 'Bleeding from the back passage' section (p. 26).

Melaena This is jet-black, tarry poo which usually smells disgusting. It is caused by blood which has been altered as it has passed through the bowel, and it means you're bleeding somewhere in your gut – from a duodenal ulcer, for example.

Treatment You need urgent medical attention, so get to casualty asap.

Medication side-effect Some medicines can change the colour of your motions. For example, iron turns them black.

Treatment Check the leaflet in the treatment pack or speak to the chemist to see if your coloured poo is a recognized side-effect of the treatment you're taking. If you're not sure, and your problem is black motions, speak to your GP to make sure it's not melaena (see above).

Hepatitis (or other similar problem) Hepatitis is inflammation of the liver, usually caused by a virus. Some types (such as hepatitis A) are caught just like tummy bugs; more serious sorts (like hepatitis B and C) are usually passed on sexually or through infected blood (e.g. sharing needles if you inject drugs). Swelling in the liver stops a pigment getting through to your bowels, so you end up with pale poo, although you're likely to notice other symptoms too – such as turning yellow (jaundice). A number of other problems can have the same effect, including some medications and gallstones.

Treatment See your GP. He'll need to run some tests to work out exactly what the problem is, and he may need to refer you to a specialist.

Malabsorption This is explained in the 'Diarrhoea' section (p. 47). Some types of malabsorption cause pale, floating motions which can be hard to flush away.

Ankle swelling

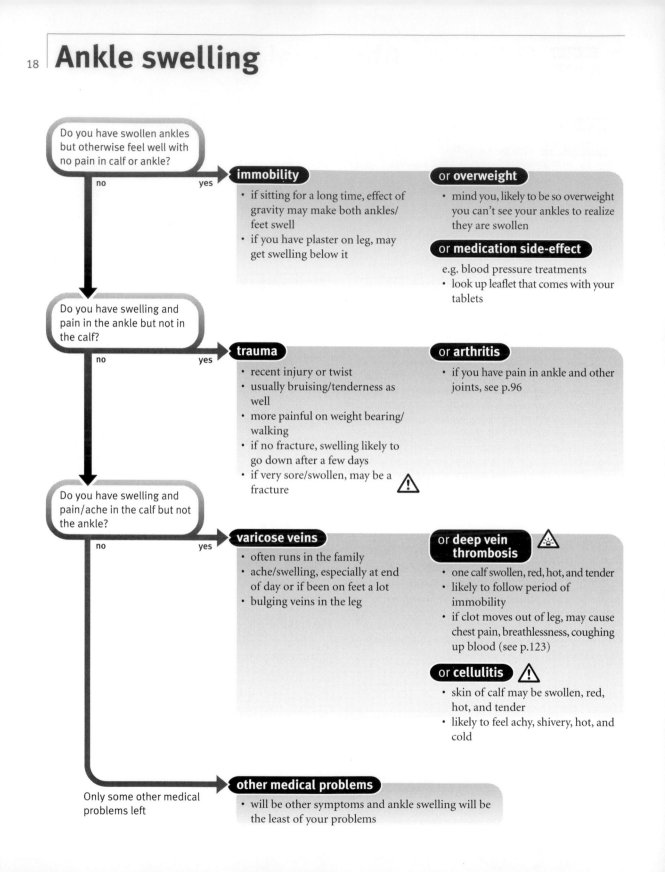

Do you have swollen ankles but otherwise feel well with no pain in calf or ankle?

no   yes

immobility
- if sitting for a long time, effect of gravity may make both ankles/feet swell
- if you have plaster on leg, may get swelling below it

or overweight
- mind you, likely to be so overweight you can't see your ankles to realize they are swollen

or medication side-effect
e.g. blood pressure treatments
- look up leaflet that comes with your tablets

Do you have swelling and pain in the ankle but not in the calf?

no   yes

trauma
- recent injury or twist
- usually bruising/tenderness as well
- more painful on weight bearing/walking
- if no fracture, swelling likely to go down after a few days
- if very sore/swollen, may be a fracture

or arthritis
- if you have pain in ankle and other joints, see p.96

Do you have swelling and pain/ache in the calf but not the ankle?

no   yes

varicose veins
- often runs in the family
- ache/swelling, especially at end of day or if been on feet a lot
- bulging veins in the leg

or deep vein thrombosis
- one calf swollen, red, hot, and tender
- likely to follow period of immobility
- if clot moves out of leg, may cause chest pain, breathlessness, coughing up blood (see p.123)

or cellulitis
- skin of calf may be swollen, red, hot, and tender
- likely to feel achy, shivery, hot, and cold

Only some other medical problems left

other medical problems
- will be other symptoms and ankle swelling will be the least of your problems

Trauma Going over on your ankle – typically during a game of footy or when staggering home from the pub – can cause a sprain or fracture. A sprain means that the ligament (the piece of gristle) attaching the outer part of your ankle to your foot is partially torn. In a fracture, part of the ankle is broken, or pulled off by the ligament. Both cause swelling as fluid escapes into the injured joint.

Treatment If the ankle is very painful or tender, there is severe swelling, or you can't take your own weight, you need to go to casualty as you may have a fracture. A sprain needs rest for a couple of days (preferably elevated on a stool), ice-packs, and a firm bandage. Painkillers or anti-inflammatory tablets (available over the counter) will relieve the pain. Then you need to get gently moving on your ankle. Some sprains take months to heal and continue to ache and swell for a while whenever you exercise. Physiotherapy and strapping may help. When the ankle feels better and you're more confident on it, you may find that running along (not up and down) a gentle slope like a beach or the camber of a road helps strengthen the joint.

Immobility If you're unable to move about much – perhaps because you're physically handicapped in some way, recovering from an injury, or on a long flight – your ankles may swell, particularly as the day goes on. This is because, as you walk, your calf muscles help your circulation by pumping the blood back up to your heart. When you're immobile, this doesn't happen, so the blood tends to pool in your legs, causing swelling.

Treatment Depending on the circumstances, there may be little you can do about this. If the swelling bothers you, keep your legs up on a stool as much as possible, and pump your calf muscles from time to time. Compression stockings – available from the chemist – can help too.

Overweight Pregnant women often get swollen ankles, because the weight of the baby partially blocks the veins returning the blood from their legs. OK, so you're not pregnant, but if you're very overweight you can experience the same problem – for baby, read excess lard.

Treatment If you're fat enough to be getting swollen ankles, you have a serious weight problem and need to shed a good few pounds. For further details, see the 'Weight gain' section.

Varicose veins These are bendy, bloated blood vessels which draw the blood back from your legs and point it in the direction of your heart. They tend to leak fluid, and this pools around the ankles. There are a number of reasons why your veins might become 'varicose' including being over-weight or suffering a previous 'deep vein thrombosis' (see below). Often, they simply run in the family.

Treatment Slim down if you're overweight. Take regular exercise and try wearing compression stockings if the swelling really bothers you. Surgery can be used for varicose veins, but they tend to come back again – discuss the situation with your GP if they're a real nuisance.

Arthritis Various types of arthritis can affect the ankles, causing painful swelling – see the 'Multiple joint pains' section (p. 88) for further details.

Medication side-effect Some prescribed treatments, such as blood pressure pills and anti-inflammatory drugs, can cause ankle swelling as a side-effect.

Treatment Look at the leaflet that comes in the pack. If it mentions swollen ankles as a possible side-effect, and the problem bothers you, discuss the situation with your GP.

Deep vein thrombosis This is explained, and the treatment outlined, in the 'Calf pain' section (p. 38).

Cellulitis This means an infection of the skin. The lower leg is a favourite site for germs getting into the skin, and the infection will result in swelling.

Treatment See your GP – this needs antibiotics.

Some other medical problem A few small print but serious diseases can make you retain fluid, leading to ankle swelling. These include kidney, liver, and bowel disease and anaemia.

Treatment Ankle swelling usually happens pretty late on in any of these diseases, so it's very unlikely that they'll come to light as a result of this symptom. If you're concerned, speak to your GP.

Arm pain

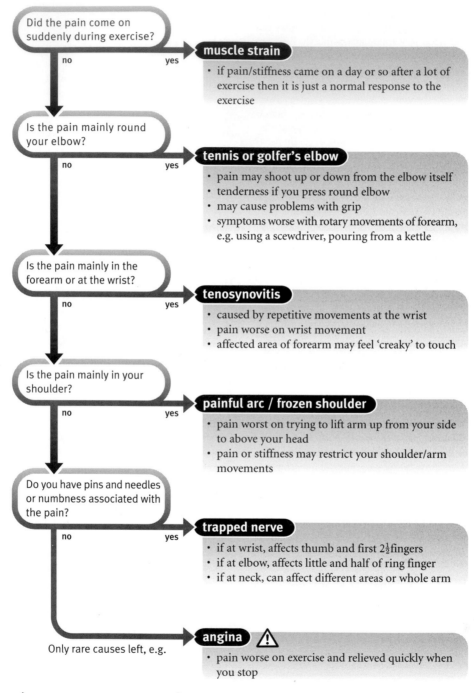

Did the pain come on suddenly during exercise?

no / yes

muscle strain
- if pain/stiffness came on a day or so after a lot of exercise then it is just a normal response to the exercise

Is the pain mainly round your elbow?

no / yes

tennis or golfer's elbow
- pain may shoot up or down from the elbow itself
- tenderness if you press round elbow
- may cause problems with grip
- symptoms worse with rotary movements of forearm, e.g. using a scewdriver, pouring from a kettle

Is the pain mainly in the forearm or at the wrist?

no / yes

tenosynovitis
- caused by repetitive movements at the wrist
- pain worse on wrist movement
- affected area of forearm may feel 'creaky' to touch

Is the pain mainly in your shoulder?

no / yes

painful arc / frozen shoulder
- pain worst on trying to lift arm up from your side to above your head
- pain or stiffness may restrict your shoulder/arm movements

Do you have pins and needles or numbness associated with the pain?

no / yes

trapped nerve
- if at wrist, affects thumb and first 2½ fingers
- if at elbow, affects little and half of ring finger
- if at neck, can affect different areas or whole arm

Only rare causes left, e.g.

angina ⚠
- pain worse on exercise and relieved quickly when you stop

Remember: ⚠ means see your GP sharpish; ⚠ means an urgent hospital job

Muscle strain The arm contains a variety of muscles, any of which are easily strained (in other words, over-stretched or partially torn) by, for example, lifting a heavy weight or injuring yourself during sport.

Treatment A mild strain doesn't need any treatment at all and will heal itself in a day or two. A more severe strain needs rest for a few days, an ice-pack (such as a bag of frozen peas wrapped in a towel) on the injured part, and some painkillers or anti-inflammatories (such as ibuprofen, which is available over the counter).

Tennis and golfer's elbow A variety of muscles help you to move your hand at the wrist. Many of these are attached to the elbow – those which pull your hand up are connected to the outer side of the elbow and those which push it down, to the inner side. The areas where these muscles attach can become inflamed – often for no reason, but sometimes through an injury or repeated use in sport – causing tennis elbow (outer side) or golfer's elbow (inner side). You don't have to play golf or tennis to suffer from these problems.

Treatment The problem burns itself out, but can take months. Heat treatment (such as a hot water bottle or heat lamp), gentle massage, a support bandage, and anti-inflammatory drugs like ibuprofen may help. If it's showing no sign of improvement and it's a real nuisance, a cortisone injection may cure it – your GP may do this for you, or refer you on to a specialist. If you do play a club or racquet sport, get some advice about your technique or grip size – minor alterations may solve the problem.

Tenosynovitis Tendons are tough cords which connect muscles to bone. They have a cling-film type sheath to help them run smoothly over each other. Repeated movements or exercise which is unusual for you can make these sheaths swell, rub, and become painful. This is tenosynovitis, and it happens most commonly at the wrist.

Treatment When it's caused by exercise you're unaccustomed to, it usually goes away on its own after a few days. Tenosynovitis caused by repetitive movements is more of a problem. Wrist supports, heat, and anti-inflammatories, as for tennis and golfer's elbow, may help; cortisone injections into the tendon sheath can also be very effective, although you'll probably have to see a specialist for this type of treatment. It's important to sort out whatever's causing it. For example, repetitive work with tools, or long hours at the keyboard without breaks or in an awkward position, may

stop the inflamed tendon sheaths from healing. Try to make some simple alterations to your work habits to solve the problem, or discuss the situation with your employer.

Painful arc/frozen shoulder A large cuff of muscles is used in moving your shoulder. If this becomes inflamed – usually for no obvious reason – the shoulder becomes sore and its movements may be restricted. This is known as 'painful arc'. In really severe cases, the pain gets so bad that movement of the shoulder is virtually reduced to zero and the joint is described as being 'frozen'.

Treatment Most of the treatments already discussed for other arm problems will help painful arc, such as heat and anti-inflammatories from the chemist. It's very important to keep the shoulder moving so it doesn't stiffen up too much. One easy way is to do an exercise in which you bend forward slightly and gently swing the arm, at the shoulder, like a pendulum, increasing the movements a little each day. Painful arc and frozen shoulder can take many months – or even a year or two – to settle. Again, a cortisone injection often helps – your GP will be able to arrange this for you. Sometimes, physiotherapy, or even surgery in really severe cases, is the answer, so discuss the situation with your GP if you're getting nowhere.

Trapped nerve The nerves leave the spinal cord, pass through the bones of the neck, and travel through various nooks and crannies before reaching their destinations in the arms. At any point in this journey, they can become trapped. Common areas include the neck, the elbow, and the wrist, and the result is pain and pins and needles or numbness.

Treatment Most trapped nerves free themselves within a day or two. If the problem lasts longer, try anti-inflammatories and gentle exercise. And if this doesn't sort it out, or the problem is severe or quickly getting worse, speak to your GP. The treatment will vary according to where exactly the nerve is trapped, but may involve painkillers, splints, cortisone injections, manipulations – and, in occasional persistent and troublesome cases, surgery.

(Angina) This is explained in the 'Chest pain' section (p. 40). Occasionally, the pain is felt in the left arm as well as – or instead of – in the chest. But remember that it's very unlikely to be the cause of arm pain in the under 45s.

Treatment See the 'Chest pain' section (p. 40).

Back pain

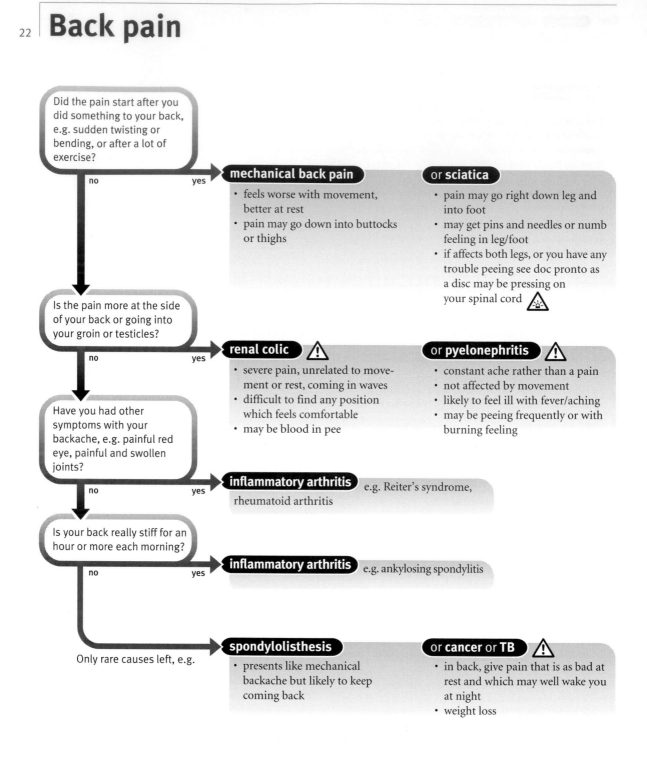

Did the pain start after you did something to your back, e.g. sudden twisting or bending, or after a lot of exercise?

no   yes →

mechanical back pain
- feels worse with movement, better at rest
- pain may go down into buttocks or thighs

or sciatica
- pain may go right down leg and into foot
- may get pins and needles or numb feeling in leg/foot
- if affects both legs, or you have any trouble peeing see doc pronto as a disc may be pressing on your spinal cord

Is the pain more at the side of your back or going into your groin or testicles?

no   yes →

renal colic
- severe pain, unrelated to movement or rest, coming in waves
- difficult to find any position which feels comfortable
- may be blood in pee

or pyelonephritis
- constant ache rather than a pain
- not affected by movement
- likely to feel ill with fever/aching
- may be peeing frequently or with burning feeling

Have you had other symptoms with your backache, e.g. painful red eye, painful and swollen joints?

no   yes →

inflammatory arthritis e.g. Reiter's syndrome, rheumatoid arthritis

Is your back really stiff for an hour or more each morning?

no   yes →

inflammatory arthritis e.g. ankylosing spondylitis

Only rare causes left, e.g. →

spondylolisthesis
- presents like mechanical backache but likely to keep coming back

or cancer or TB
- in back, give pain that is as bad at rest and which may well wake you at night
- weight loss

Remember: ⚠ means see your GP sharpish; ⚠ means an urgent hospital job

Back pain

Mechanical back pain The back is made up of so many interlocking bits and pieces (muscles, bones, joints, discs, ligaments, and tendons), that it's pretty much impossible for the doc to be totally specific about which bit you've strained or inflamed. And it really doesn't matter anyway, because they're all treated in much the same way – so they're lumped together under the blanket term, 'mechanical back pain'.

Treatment The days of strict bed rest are long gone. There are two main areas to focus on. First, relieve the pain. The chemist can help with painkillers: anti-inflammatory drugs (e.g. ibuprofen) or paracetamol/codeine mixtures are usually effective. Heat and massage may also help ease the pain, especialy if you have a lot of spasm – a cramp-type contraction of the muscles of your back. Second, get your back moving. Getting up and about, so long as you avoid heavy lifting, twisting, and so on, will help your back heal, even if it makes it feel a bit more painful to begin with. Going swimming is ideal exercise. And stay optimistic: whatever treatment you have, you've an 80–90% chance of the problem being better within six to eight weeks. It's important to get back to work as soon as possible, even if your back doesn't feel 100%. If you're not noticing any signs of improvement after a week or two, consider seeing an osteopath as manipulation may speed things up. And don't expect your doctor to arrange an X-ray of your back, as it's very unlikely to help.

If you get repeated episodes of mechanical pain, then try some preventive measures. These include: dieting if you're overweight; doing gentle back exercises and swimming regularly; being careful with your posture and with lifting; and using a firm mattress.

Sciatica Between each bone which makes up the vertebral column is a shock absorber known as an intervertebral disc. If one of these shifts sideways, or leaks some fluid, it can irritate a nearby nerve – commonly the sciatic nerve, which runs down the back of your leg. Hence, 'sciatica' or 'slipped disc'.

Treatment Much the same as for mechanical pain. As the pain can be quite severe, though, you may need something prescribed by your GP if over-the-counter medicines aren't strong enough. Very occasionally, the problem doesn't settle down or the nerve is quite badly damaged, in which case your GP is likely to refer you to an orthopaedic surgeon (bone specialist) to see if surgery might help.

Very rarely a slipped disc can press on the spinal cord giving pain down both legs and trouble peeing. This is an urgent hospital job.

Renal colic This is a stone (usually like a small piece of gravel) in the tube joining the kidney to the bladder. This tube is very thin and muscular, and squeezes hard to push the stone through, causing horrendous pain.

Treatment It probably depends who it's quickest to get to – the local hospital or your GP. You'll be in so much pain you won't really care who sees you, you'll just want it sorted out asap. It needs strong painkillers, usually by injection, and a high fluid intake. If your GP does treat you, he may need to send you to hospital anyway if it doesn't quickly settle down. And one way or another, if it's your first attack, you're likely to need further tests.

Inflammatory arthritis Arthritis means worn down or inflamed joints. Young or youngish men occasionally suffer from a type of arthritis which causes a distinct pattern of pain in certain joints (including the back) and which can cause problems elsewhere (e.g. the eye and skin). This is 'inflammatory arthritis' and it comes in various forms (including rheumatoid arthritis, Reiter's syndrome, and ankylosing spondylitis – each of these vary in terms of their cause and how they affect you. For more information, see the 'Multiple joint pain' section, p. 89).

Treatment Your GP is very likely to refer you to a consultant rheumatologist (a joint specialist) as you will probably need specialized drug treatment. It's very important to keep as active as possible and to follow a lot of the guidance outlined above for mechanical back pain.

Pyelonephritis An infection of the kidney.

Treatment Drink plenty of fluids and see your GP – you will need a course of antibiotics. This problem is quite unusual in young men, so you may also need some tests on your kidney to see why you've developed this infection. Your own doc may do this or he may refer you to hospital.

Spondylolisthesis This is a shift forward of one of the bones of the vertebral column on the one underneath.

Treatment Most just require painkillers and the usual back advice outlined above. If the shift is large, or the pain prolonged and severe, then surgery may be the only answer.

Rare serious causes There's a whole heap of small print stuff, including cancers and bone infection, which can cause back pain. Fortunately, they're all incredibly rare.

Treatment If you think you have a rare serious cause, according to the flow chart, see your GP. If he thinks so too – unlikely – he'll arrange tests or a specialist's opinion.

Bad breath

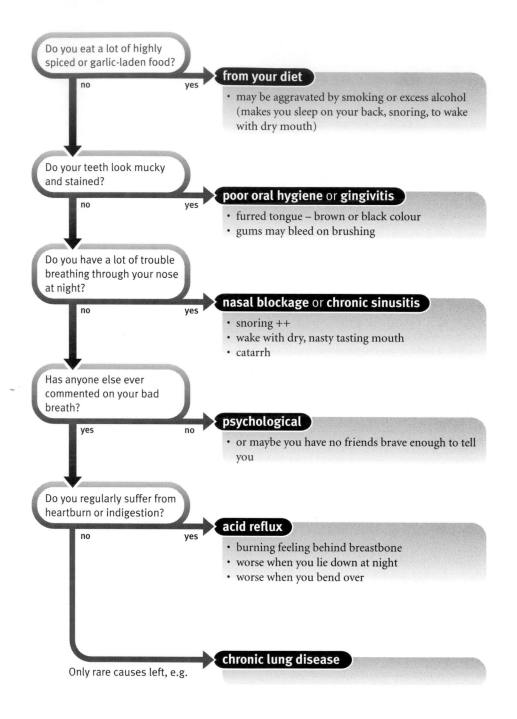

Do you eat a lot of highly spiced or garlic-laden food?

no / yes

from your diet
- may be aggravated by smoking or excess alcohol (makes you sleep on your back, snoring, to wake with dry mouth)

Do your teeth look mucky and stained?

no / yes

poor oral hygiene or gingivitis
- furred tongue – brown or black colour
- gums may bleed on brushing

Do you have a lot of trouble breathing through your nose at night?

no / yes

nasal blockage or chronic sinusitis
- snoring ++
- wake with dry, nasty tasting mouth
- catarrh

Has anyone else ever commented on your bad breath?

yes / no

psychological
- or maybe you have no friends brave enough to tell you

Do you regularly suffer from heartburn or indigestion?

no / yes

acid reflux
- burning feeling behind breastbone
- worse when you lie down at night
- worse when you bend over

Only rare causes left, e.g.

chronic lung disease

Bad breath

Poor oral hygiene Mouth neglect is far and away the most common cause of persistent dog-breath ('halitosis'). Unsavoury muck collecting around your teeth and gums – or on your tongue – festers, releasing a smell.

Treatment Regular brushing and flossing will help prevent your mouth turning into, and smelling like, a dustbin. But don't forget your tongue, because a dirty tongue is basically a swamp of microscopic bits of decaying food. A little known trick involves scrubbing the tongue regularly with a soft toothbrush. Push it forward as you do this, or you'll retch and rather spoil the effect. Mouthwashes and breath fresheners may help, but remember they're only cosmetic and don't get to the root of the problem. Saliva is a natural mouthwash which you can stimulate by chewing gum (sugar-free, of course). Also, drink plenty of fluids and swill your mouth with water regularly to dislodge any stuck food particles.

Diet You don't need a medical degree to realize that last night's vindaloo or chicken kiev may put people off entering your personal space for a day or two.

Treatment You could avoid curries and highly spiced foods, but then life would hardly be worth living, would it? It's more realistic just to put up with the problem until your breath is sweet smelling again after a day or so – or use breath fresheners or mouthwashes to camouflage the problem. And count your mouth's blessings – the smell isn't half as bad as the odour coming out the other end.

Gingivitis This means infected gums and is usually caused by poor oral hygiene, as outlined above.

Treatment This needs a mouthwash or antibiotics, which your dentist can provide. He ought to give your teeth the once-over anyway, as you've probably been neglecting them, and can give you advice on how to keep your teeth and gums healthy in the future.

Nasal blockage or chronic sinusitis Anything which permanently blocks your nose – such as hay fever, a constantly runny nose, polyps, or a bent nose from a previous injury – will make you snore and breathe through your mouth (see the 'Blocked nose' section, p. 31). As a result, your mouth tends to dry out and this, in turn, causes bad breath. Chronic sinusitis is explained in the 'Hoarse voice' section. The dripping of catarrh down the back of the throat can cause bad breath, especially if the catarrh contains certain types of germs.

Treatment If you have to breath through your mouth all the time because your nose is stuffed up, then you have to sort out whatever's causing the blockage if you want to cure your bad breath. This means a trip to your GP. You'll probably end up with either nose sprays or an appointment with an Ear, Nose, and Throat ('ENT') surgeon for possible surgery. A course of antibiotics may help chronic sinusitis – but usually only for a while. Again, it's a question of sorting out your blocked nose (as in the 'Chronic sinusitis' part of the 'Hoarse voice' section, p. 67), otherwise it's likely to keep coming back.

Psychological You might find that the problem is more in your mind than in your mouth. Some people are simply self-conscious, and become very aware of minor problems with their breath which others would accept as normal. This is just an aspect of their personality and doesn't usually cause a great problem. But if you are depressed or suffering from severe anxiety, you might focus on your breath, becoming convinced that it stinks, despite the fact that no one else ever notices a problem.

Treatment If you think it's possible you're just worrying unnecessarily, your best bet is simply to ask someone who you can trust to give you a straight answer. At least you'll then know whether you've been worrying over nothing, or whether you've got a problem, which you can then get sorted out as described above. If you're suffering badly with anxiety, or you – or friends or family – think you might be depressed, then follow the advice given in the 'Feeling tense' (p. 59) and 'Feeling down' (p. 57) sections.

Acid reflux This is explained, and the treatment outlined, in the 'Indigestion' section (p. 71). Acid, and the stomach contents, coming up into the gullet can release a smell causing bad breath.

Lung disease Any lung disease which produces a lot of infected catarrh can cause bad breath, simply because you'll keep coughing up foul-smelling phlegm. This is very rarely the cause of halitosis, though – especially if your chest isn't really giving you major problems.

Treatment See your GP to get the lung trouble sorted out.

Bleeding from the back passage

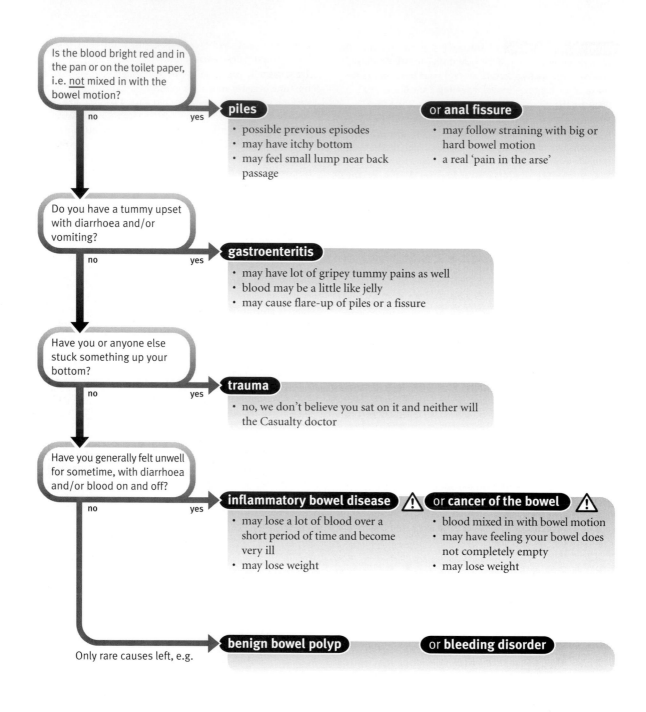

Is the blood bright red and in the pan or on the toilet paper, i.e. <u>not</u> mixed in with the bowel motion?

no   yes

piles
- possible previous episodes
- may have itchy bottom
- may feel small lump near back passage

or anal fissure
- may follow straining with big or hard bowel motion
- a real 'pain in the arse'

Do you have a tummy upset with diarrhoea and/or vomiting?

no   yes

gastroenteritis
- may have lot of gripey tummy pains as well
- blood may be a little like jelly
- may cause flare-up of piles or a fissure

Have you or anyone else stuck something up your bottom?

no   yes

trauma
- no, we don't believe you sat on it and neither will the Casualty doctor

Have you generally felt unwell for sometime, with diarrhoea and/or blood on and off?

no   yes

inflammatory bowel disease ⚠
- may lose a lot of blood over a short period of time and become very ill
- may lose weight

or cancer of the bowel ⚠
- blood mixed in with bowel motion
- may have feeling your bowel does not completely empty
- may lose weight

Only rare causes left, e.g.

benign bowel polyp

or bleeding disorder

Remember: ⚠ means see your GP sharpish; ⚠ means an urgent hospital job

Bleeding from the back passage

Piles These are varicose veins (swollen veins full of blood) in your back passage. They are usually caused by constipation – straining when you go to the toilet tends to make the veins swell. They often leak some blood, which you'll notice in the toilet or on the paper when you wipe yourself. They aren't usually painful unless they strangulate – this means that they're being throttled by the muscle of your anus, causing severe pain, increased swelling, and more bleeding.

Treatment Piles will often sort themselves out, especially if you can avoid straining when you go to the toilet. Constipation is usually helped by increasing your fibre and fluid intake, and doing more physical exercise. You can kick-start the process by using a laxative from the chemist, but these are probably best kept to a minimum. It's also important not to spend too long in the khazi, as the posture of sitting on the toilet actually makes the problem worse – so no reading while you're in there. And don't ignore the early morning urge to open your bowels, no matter how pushed you are for time. Creams from the chemist will help any irritation the piles are causing, but will make no difference to the bleeding. If you keep getting problems, see your GP – he may refer you to a surgeon for a small operation which should solve the problem. You'll need urgent treatment if your piles have strangulated. The pain will normally get you to your GP pretty quickly.

Anal fissure This is a split in the back passage. Again, constipation is the likely cause; straining to pass a large motion causes the split, which then leaks some blood. It can also start after an attack of diarrhoea.

Treatment Most fissures heal themselves quickly. The advice already given about constipation (see above) is vital. Fissures are painful, so it's tempting to avoid going to the toilet. If you do this, you'll get more constipated, with the risk of opening up the split again when you do go – so get those bowels opening regularly and easily. Keep the tail end clean to give the fissure a chance to heal: carry around a small pack of wet-wipes so you can clean up thoroughly and painlessly each time you go to the toilet. Creams from the chemist usually help ease the pain. If you seem to be getting nowhere, see your GP – he can prescribe alternative creams or refer you to a surgeon for a small operation if all else fails.

Gastroenteritis This is explained in the 'Abdominal pain' (p. 13) and 'Diarrhoea' (p. 47) sections. One particular germ – 'campylobacter' – can inflame the bowel so much that it causes bleeding.

Treatment See the 'Abdominal pain' section. If the bleeding happens a few times, it's worth contacting your GP. He may want to check you out for the Campylobacter germ, because antibiotics may get you better quicker.

Trauma Nature did not intend anything to be poked up the backside. It's not surprising, then, that sticking objects in your rear end can cause some damage, resulting in bleeding – and if you've ever spoken to anyone who's worked in a casualty department, you'd be surprised how often this type of problem is seen, although some of these stories are probably urban legends. Homosexuals who indulge in anal sex are obviously prone to this type of trauma – but the greater risk in this situation lies in transmitting infections.

Treatment Unless the bleeding is very insignificant and painless, it's best to get to casualty to check how much damage has been done (and to add to their stock of stories).

Inflammatory bowel disease This is explained, and the treatment outlined, in the 'Diarrhoea' section (p. 47).

Cancer This is very unlikely in the under 40s. For further details, see the 'Diarrhoea' section (p. 47).

Rare causes A few rarities like polyps in the bowel (which sometimes run in families) and bleeding disorders (problems with your blood clotting) can cause bleeding from the back passage.

Treatment See your GP – if he thinks you might have a rare problem like this, he'll get it checked out.

Blisters

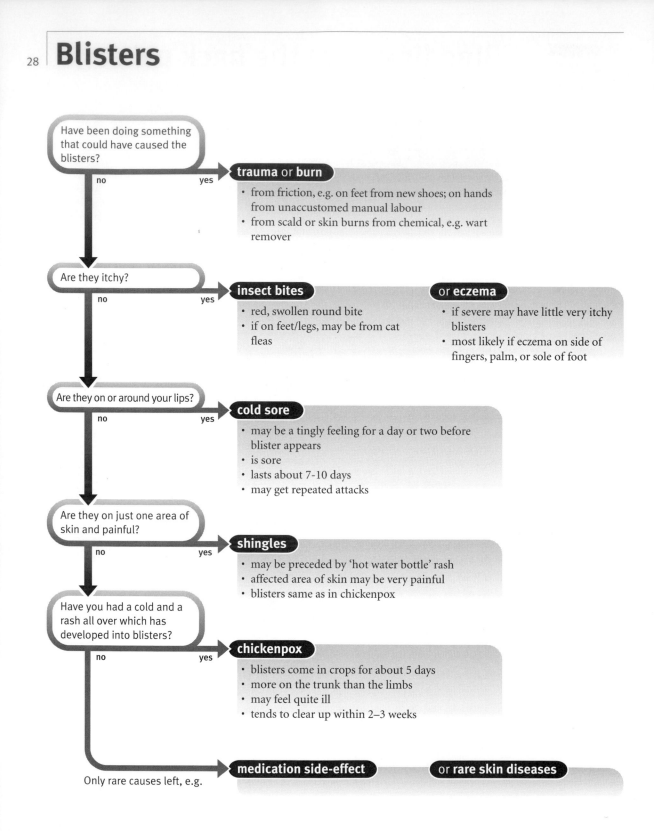

Have been doing something that could have caused the blisters?

no   yes

trauma or burn

- from friction, e.g. on feet from new shoes; on hands from unaccustomed manual labour
- from scald or skin burns from chemical, e.g. wart remover

Are they itchy?

no   yes

insect bites

- red, swollen round bite
- if on feet/legs, may be from cat fleas

or eczema

- if severe may have little very itchy blisters
- most likely if eczema on side of fingers, palm, or sole of foot

Are they on or around your lips?

no   yes

cold sore

- may be a tingly feeling for a day or two before blister appears
- is sore
- lasts about 7-10 days
- may get repeated attacks

Are they on just one area of skin and painful?

no   yes

shingles

- may be preceded by 'hot water bottle' rash
- affected area of skin may be very painful
- blisters same as in chickenpox

Have you had a cold and a rash all over which has developed into blisters?

no   yes

chickenpox

- blisters come in crops for about 5 days
- more on the trunk than the limbs
- may feel quite ill
- tends to clear up within 2–3 weeks

Only rare causes left, e.g.

medication side-effect

or rare skin diseases

Trauma Everyone is familiar with blisters on the feet caused by new shoes or a long walk or run. The cause is friction, which leads to a build-up of fluid under the skin. Similar blisters can also develop after a burn.

Treatment Friction blisters settle down quickly and don't need any treatment except maybe a change of shoe and a protective plaster. A burn may take longer to heal – if you're worried, get it checked by the nurse at your practice to make sure it doesn't need any special dressings or antibiotics. Usually, it's better to leave blisters alone rather than deliberately burst them.

Insect bites These are discussed, and their treatment outlined, in the 'Itchy skin' section (p. 77). They can sometimes result in quite large blisters. If you keep getting problems with insect bites, try to work out – and sort out – wherever they're coming from. Likely sources include pets (dogs, cats, and birds) and bedding or furniture.

Cold sore See the 'Rash on the face' section (p. 119).

Eczema One type of eczema – 'pompholyx' – can cause tiny, itchy blisters on the palms and sides of the fingers. The same pattern can also develop on the feet. Other forms of eczema can also develop blisters when they're flaring up or infected. For more information on eczema, see the 'Itchy skin' section.

Treatment Mild pompholyx may be helped by a moisturizer and hydrocortisone 1% cream from the chemist. It's important to avoid things which might irritate your skin such as detergents and strong soaps. Often, though, this problem will need stronger treatments, in which case your GP can help. You'll also need to see him if you have any other type of eczema which has flared up so badly that it's caused blisters.

Shingles Once you've had chickenpox, the virus which causes it never fully leaves your system – it lies dormant somewhere in your spine. In the future, for no obvious reason, it can reactivate, resulting in shingles.

Treatment Shingles goes away on its own over a few weeks. The blisters become weepy, then scab over, and finally heal. Usually, the only treatment needed is nothing more than painkillers and dressings from the chemist. It's worth steering clear of women who are (or are trying to get) pregnant while you have the rash. This is because, when you have shingles, it's possible to pass the germ on to anyone who's never had chickenpox before, and this can damage a developing baby – although the risk is very small.

There are lots of old wives' tales about shingles, but they're all nonsense. The only times it can really be troublesome are if you already have some problem which weakens your immune system (such as being on high-dose steroid tablets or chemotherapy drugs for cancer) or if shingles affects the area around your eye (it can get into the eye itself, causing complications). In both cases, contact your GP urgently.

Some doctors prescribe a certain type of medication in shingles, but this is only really useful in the elderly or in the special situations outlined above – and then only if started very soon after the rash first appears. Occasionally, the pain of shingles can carry on long after the rash has gone – this is known as post-herpetic neuralgia. Again, this only usually affects the elderly. It can be treated quite effectively, so if you think you have this problem, discuss the situation with your GP.

Chickenpox Viruses can cause all sorts of rashes (as well as other typical symptoms like a fever and sore throat) – sometimes these result in blisters, the most well-known example being chickenpox.

Treatment Usually, these viruses don't require any special treatment other than the paracetamol and fluids you'd normally take for a cold or flu. If you get chickenpox, you may feel pretty unwell – rest, and use calamine lotion to ease the itch. You'll need to contact your GP if you already have a weakened immune system (see the 'Shingles' section above) or if you're becoming increasingly unwell, especially if you develop a bad cough or breathlessness (the virus can occasionally affect the lungs). The advice given in the 'Shingles' section about avoiding pregnant women applies too.

Medication side-effect Some prescribed treatments can cause blisters as a side-effect, though it's pretty unlikely that you'll be taking any of them.

Treatment If you think your blisters might be caused by your medication, discuss the situation with whoever prescribed them.

Rare skin disorders Some very small print skin diseases can cause unexplained blisters which may keep coming back.

Treatment See your GP – if he thinks you've got an unusual skin disease, he'll arrange for you to see a dermatologist (a skin specialist).

Blocked nose

Is this a short-term problem associated with sneezing, a runny nose, and a bit of a sore throat?

no / **yes**

a cold
- blocked nose, especially at night

Do you tend to get blocked up in the summer?

no / **yes**

hayfever
- also sneezing; runny nose; itchy, runny eyes
- may be worse at certain times in the summer, depending on whether you are allergic to grass or tree pollen
- may get some asthma in the summer as well

Do you get worse or only get symptoms in certain situations, e.g. if dusting or making beds; near animals?

no / **yes**

other types of allergic rhinitis
- if worse in morning or if dusting/bed-making then allergy to house dust mite
- may be allergy to cats, dogs, horses
- can get all the hayfever symptoms, including asthma

Is your nose blocked virtually all the time?

no / **yes**

nasal polyps
- may feel there is something blocking your nostril
- lose sense of smell/decreased sense of taste
- may talk 'nasally'
- likely to get sinus trouble with colds

or septal deviation
- may be result of injury to nose
- in itself does not cause sneezing, runny nose
- likely to get sinus trouble with colds
- likely to get nose bleeds

or vasomotor rhinitis
- blocked with loads of watery mucus being produced

Do you snort cocaine?

no / **yes**

cocaine use
- nasal problems are a well known side-effect

Only rare causes left, e.g.

medication side-effect
- look up the leaflet with your medicine

or septal haematoma
- result of serious bang to the nose
- feels suddenly and totally blocked

Blocked nose

A cold Your nose reacts to the virus which causes colds by making more snot (or, to get technical, 'mucus') to prevent any more germs getting into your system. The result: the familiar bunged-up nose.

Treatment There's no point seeing your GP about a cold because there's no magic cure. Just take plenty of fluids and paracetamol for the headache or sore throat which goes with the cold. The stuffed-up feeling may be helped by steam inhalations.

Hay fever This is an allergy to pollen, which inflames the inside of your nose and throat. The glands in your nose go into overdrive, producing loads of mucus, which results in a runny, blocked nose and sneezing.

Treatment Simple measures include avoiding long walks when the pollen count is high (usually early morning and evening), and keeping the car windows wound up (otherwise the car acts as a pollen trap). Further advice about eye problems caused by hay fever are given in the 'Red eye' section (p. 121). Have a word with your chemist – a lot of effective hay fever treatment is now available over the counter, including antihistamine tablets and steroid nose sprays. If you're getting nowhere, see your GP. He may try other antihistamines or nose sprays, or, if you're really bad, he may even use steroids in the form of a course of tablets or a 'one-off' injection.

Other types of allergic rhinitis You may be allergic to something other than pollen, resulting in stuffy-nosed misery very similar to hay fever ('rhinitis'). Your symptoms may only happen in specific situations (e.g. cat allergy) or may be there much of the time (e.g. house dust mite allergy).

Treatment If you can, avoid whatever you're allergic to. Allergy tests aren't usually much help – it's either obvious what the allergy is, or, if not, then it's usually something you can't really avoid anyway (such as house dust – although, in this case, bear in mind that feather pillows act as a dust trap, so using foam ones may help). Effective treatments like antihistamines and steroid nose sprays are available from the chemist.

Vasomotor rhinitis This makes your nose produce loads of watery snot which can leak out like water from a tap. It's possibly caused by leaky blood vessels in the nose.

Treatment Steroid nose sprays are worth a try, although they may not work as well as in the allergic types of rhinitis. Otherwise, see your GP, who may prescribe other types of nose spray. Surgery can be considered if you're really desperate.

Nasal polyps These are fleshy bits of gristle which can grow inside your nose, blocking the airway. They are more common in people with allergic rhinitis or asthma.

Treatment Steroid nose sprays from the chemist can shrink polyps down enough to ease the block. If you're getting nowhere and you'd consider surgery, see your GP, who may refer you to an Ear, Nose, and Throat ('ENT') specialist – polyps can be cut out, although they can come back again in the future.

Cocaine use Sniffing up naughty substances can cause some damage, leading to a drippy and blocked nose.

Treatment Easy – avoid snorting cocaine.

Septal deviation The nasal septum is the bony bit in the middle of your nose separating your two nostrils. It can bend to one side or the other, causing a blockage. This is usually the result of an old injury – or maybe you were born with it.

Treatment The only way to cure this is with surgery. So if the problem is bad enough, speak to your GP, who will refer you to an ENT surgeon.

Medication side-effect Some treatments – either prescribed or over-the-counter – can cause a blocked nose. For example, certain types of spray used for blocked noses and sinusitis (available from the chemist) cause a 'rebound' effect: this means they help while you use them, but, when you stop, the stuffiness can return worse than it was in the first place. As a result, some people end up using the spray constantly, because the problem gets much worse whenever they stop. Some blood pressure and prostate pills prescribed by your doc also have the side-effect of causing a blocked-up nose.

Treatment If you think an over-the-counter spray may be making you worse, speak to your chemist or GP. And if you're on prescribed treatment, check the leaflet in the pack – if a blocked or runny nose is mentioned as a side-effect, see your GP, as he may be able to stop the treatment or prescribe you something else instead.

Septal haematoma This is a large bruise of the nasal septum (see above). The internal swelling it causes is so large that it blocks the nose. It's rare, but occasionally results from a serious thump on the nose.

Treatment Go to casualty. The blood which causes the internal swelling needs to be drained off, otherwise your nose can end up with permanent damage.

Blood in sperm

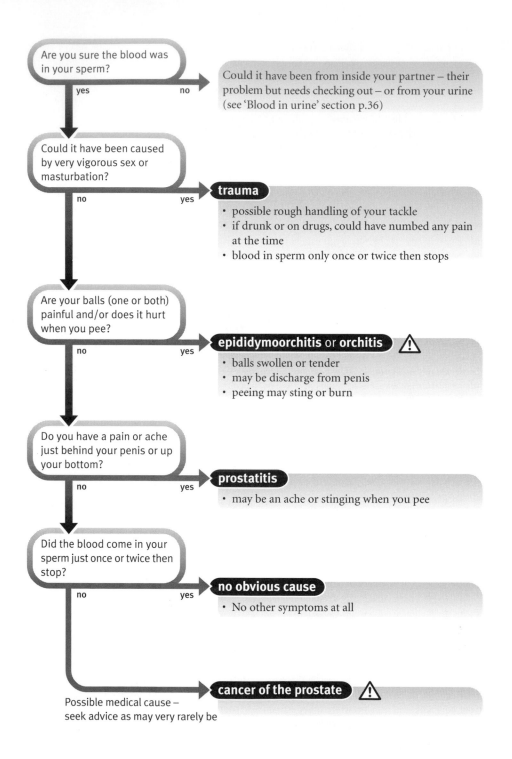

Are you sure the blood was in your sperm?

yes · no

Could it have been from inside your partner – their problem but needs checking out – or from your urine (see 'Blood in urine' section p.36)

Could it have been caused by very vigorous sex or masturbation?

no · yes

trauma
- possible rough handling of your tackle
- if drunk or on drugs, could have numbed any pain at the time
- blood in sperm only once or twice then stops

Are your balls (one or both) painful and/or does it hurt when you pee?

no · yes

epididymoorchitis or **orchitis**
- balls swollen or tender
- may be discharge from penis
- peeing may sting or burn

Do you have a pain or ache just behind your penis or up your bottom?

no · yes

prostatitis
- may be an ache or stinging when you pee

Did the blood come in your sperm just once or twice then stop?

no · yes

no obvious cause
- No other symptoms at all

cancer of the prostate

Possible medical cause – seek advice as may very rarely be

Trauma There are lots of blood vessels in the penis, testicles, and spermatic cord (the tube which carries the sperm from the testicles to the penis). If one is damaged, it will leak a little blood which will then appear in the sperm. The likeliest causes are very vigorous sex or masturbation.

Treatment Once you've got over the quite considerable shock of seeing blood in your sperm, there's nothing to do but wait and see. When trauma is the cause it's almost always a one-off, and it causes no harm at all – so you'll soon be able to forget about it.

No obvious cause Usually, no reason is found for blood in the sperm, even if it keeps happening and you have it thoroughly checked out – in men under the age of 40 with this symptom, tests show a cause in only 20% of cases.

Treatment In most men, the problem usually clears up on its own within a month. If it hasn't it's worth going to see your GP. He may check you out himself, or refer you on for tests – this is more to make sure there's no serious problem rather than find a specific cause.

Epididymoorchitis or orchitis These are fully explained in the 'Pain in the testicle' (p. 101) and 'Swelling in the groin' (p. 131) sections.

Prostatitis The prostate gland is the size of a small walnut and sits at the base of the bladder, with the tube which carries urine (the urethra) going right through it. It produces some of the fluid which makes up sperm. If a germ infects the gland, it causes swelling and pain, and it can leak blood into the sperm – this is called acute prostatitis. The germ is sometimes, though not always, sexually transmitted. Occasionally, the germ can stay in the prostate a long time and cause repeated or persistent trouble ('chronic prostatitis').

Treatment See your doctor. He'll probably need to examine you – including the infamous finger in the bottom routine (he can feel the prostate gland through your back passage). If he thinks you have prostatitis, you'll need antibiotics, usually for a few weeks (maybe even longer for chronic prostatitis). And if the cause might be a sexually transmitted germ, he may send you to a clinic for further tests – mainly to make sure you don't have any other similar germs which might need treatment. The clinic may want to test your partner too.

Rare medical causes A few highly unlikely problems can cause blood in the sperm. These range from TB to cancer of the prostate.

Treatment If you think your pattern of symptoms puts you into one of these categories, you're probably wrong, but get yourself checked by your GP.

Blood in spit

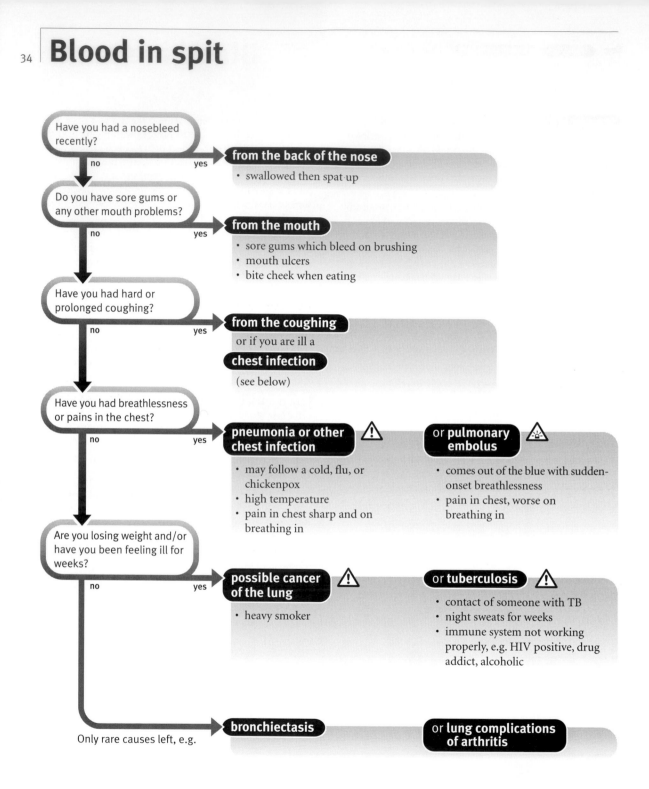

Have you had a nosebleed recently?

no   yes

from the back of the nose
- swallowed then spat up

Do you have sore gums or any other mouth problems?

no   yes

from the mouth
- sore gums which bleed on brushing
- mouth ulcers
- bite cheek when eating

Have you had hard or prolonged coughing?

no   yes

from the coughing

or if you are ill a

chest infection

(see below)

Have you had breathlessness or pains in the chest?

no   yes

pneumonia or other chest infection ⚠
- may follow a cold, flu, or chickenpox
- high temperature
- pain in chest sharp and on breathing in

or pulmonary embolus ⚠
- comes out of the blue with sudden-onset breathlessness
- pain in chest, worse on breathing in

Are you losing weight and/or have you been feeling ill for weeks?

no   yes

possible cancer of the lung ⚠
- heavy smoker

or tuberculosis ⚠
- contact of someone with TB
- night sweats for weeks
- immune system not working properly, e.g. HIV positive, drug addict, alcoholic

Only rare causes left, e.g.

bronchiectasis

or lung complications of arthritis

Remember: ⚠ means see your GP sharpish; ⚠ means an urgent hospital job

Blood in spit

Hard or prolonged coughing If you cough long or hard enough, whatever the cause of the cough, you can rupture a small blood vessel in your windpipe. Blood will leak into your spit, which you then cough up. As the blood vessel heals up, the bleeding stops.

Treatment There's no specific treatment needed – usually the blood only appears in your phlegm once or twice before it all settles down. Otherwise, all you need to do is treat whatever's causing the cough, which is probably a virus infection of your throat and windpipe. There's no magic cure – just try steam inhalations, plenty of fluids, and avoid cigarette smoke. If you're coughing green or yellow phlegm and you feel ill, breathless, or feverish, you may need antibiotics, so discuss the situation with your GP.

From a nosebleed or from the mouth Blood from a nosebleed can drip back into the throat and then be coughed up. The same can happen to blood from the mouth (such as a cut or bleeding gums).

Treatment These situations are harmless and don't need any particular treatment.

Pneumonia A severe form of chest infection. See 'Cough' section (p. 43).

Treatment This is covered in the 'Cough' section (p. 43).

Pulmonary embolus This is a blood clot in the lung. It usually forms somewhere else in the body and is carried in the circulation to the lungs, where it blocks a blood vessel. As a result, a small part of the lung is starved of oxygen, causing pain, breathlessness, and blood in the spit. It's rare in men under 50 – very occasionally, it can be caused by blood clots forming in the leg veins, which can happen if you've not used your leg muscles for a while (e.g. during a long haul flight or when your leg's in plaster).

Treatment A definite hospital job. A bad one will leave you in no doubt what to do, because the symptoms will be severe – call an ambulance. They can be more subtle, though. If in real doubt, get advice from your GP.

Tuberculosis TB is an infection of the lung caused by a particular germ which can make you very unwell and can be difficult to treat. It is rare these days, though does sometimes occur, especially in immigrants.

Treatment Your first stop is likely to be your GP. After tests, especially an X-ray of your chest, he will refer you to the local chest consultant for specialized treatment.

Lung cancer This occurs most commonly between the ages of 50 and 75 – so younger men can relax. The blood vessels supplying the cancer can leak, causing repeated episodes of blood in the spit, which is how this type of cancer may first show itself.

Treatment As for tuberculosis – a chest X-ray will show a shadow and the specialist will arrange further tests to confirm the diagnosis, and will then plan your treatment. This is likely to involve surgery (to remove the cancer), radiotherapy (treatment with radiation rays), or chemotherapy (treatment with powerful drugs).

Other medical rarities There are a number of unusual medical conditions which can reveal themselves by causing bloodstained spit. Some affect only the lung (such as bronchiectasis – a constantly infected and damaged part of the lung) and others affect other parts of the body (such as some unusual joint diseases).

Treatment You are highly unlikely to be affected by any of these conditions – see your GP if you want the problem checked out.

Blood in urine

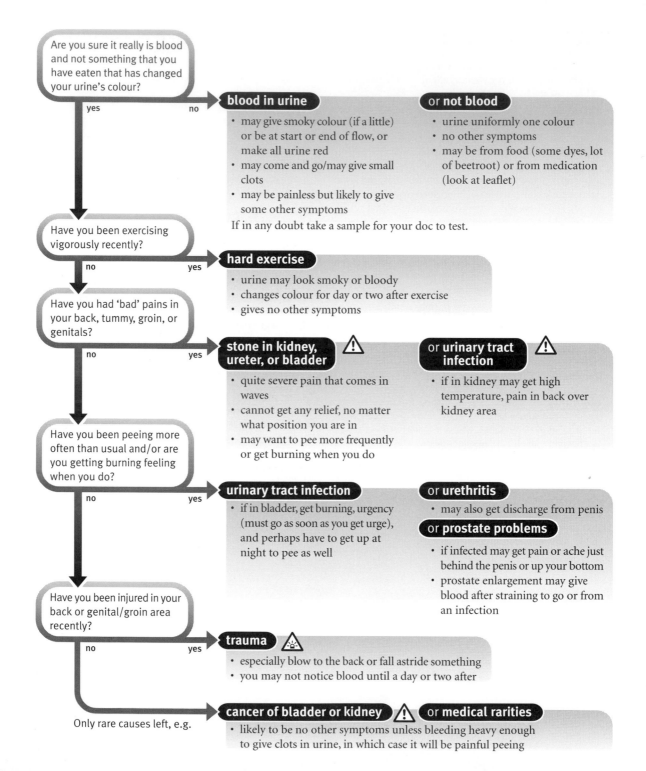

Are you sure it really is blood and not something that you have eaten that has changed your urine's colour?

yes   no

blood in urine
- may give smoky colour (if a little) or be at start or end of flow, or make all urine red
- may come and go/may give small clots
- may be painless but likely to give some other symptoms

If in any doubt take a sample for your doc to test.

or not blood
- urine uniformly one colour
- no other symptoms
- may be from food (some dyes, lot of beetroot) or from medication (look at leaflet)

Have you been exercising vigorously recently?

no   yes

hard exercise
- urine may look smoky or bloody
- changes colour for day or two after exercise
- gives no other symptoms

Have you had 'bad' pains in your back, tummy, groin, or genitals?

no   yes

stone in kidney, ureter, or bladder
- quite severe pain that comes in waves
- cannot get any relief, no matter what position you are in
- may want to pee more frequently or get burning when you do

or urinary tract infection
- if in kidney may get high temperature, pain in back over kidney area

Have you been peeing more often than usual and/or are you getting burning feeling when you do?

no   yes

urinary tract infection
- if in bladder, get burning, urgency (must go as soon as you get urge), and perhaps have to get up at night to pee as well

or urethritis
- may also get discharge from penis

or prostate problems
- if infected may get pain or ache just behind the penis or up your bottom
- prostate enlargement may give blood after straining to go or from an infection

Have you been injured in your back or genital/groin area recently?

no   yes

trauma
- especially blow to the back or fall astride something
- you may not notice blood until a day or two after

Only rare causes left, e.g.

cancer of bladder or kidney   **or medical rarities**
- likely to be no other symptoms unless bleeding heavy enough to give clots in urine, in which case it will be painful peeing

Kidney stone Stones, like bits of gravel, can develop in your kidney (which makes your urine) or your bladder (which stores it). The irritation they cause can lead to bleeding, so blood appears in your urine. This can also happen if the stone travels down the tube leading from the kidney to bladder (the 'ureter'), which is usually very painful (see the 'Renal colic' part of the 'Back pain' section, p. 23).

Treatment See the 'Back pain' (p. 23) and 'Waterworks problems' (p. 151) sections for advice on treating kidney and bladder stones.

Hard exercise A really long road-run or a tough game of footy on a hard surface can leave you 'peeing blood'. Except it isn't really blood at all. The red blood cells simply get mashed up when they pass through the blood vessels in your pounding feet. This makes them leak their pigment, which is passed out in your urine and can look just like blood.

Treatment This is harmless, so long as it doesn't keep happening whenever you exercise (in which case it can cause anaemia). But if you're not absolutely sure this is the cause, or you feel ill, you need to see a doctor – and try to take a specimen of urine for him to test.

Urinary tract infection A germ in your waterworks can inflame your kidney, bladder, or urethra (the tube you pee out of) so much that they leak blood. For further details and advice about treatment, see the 'Urinary tract infection' part of the 'Waterworks problems' section.

Urethritis A sexually transmitted germ can inflame your urethra to the point that it leaks a little blood when you pee.

Treatment See the 'Urethritis' part of the 'Penis sores and/or discharge' section (p. 107).

Prostate problems An infected or enlarged prostate gland can leak blood into the urine – either because the gland is inflamed, or because a blood vessel on the gland leaks. Further details are given in the 'Blood in sperm' (p. 33) and 'Waterworks problems' (p. 151) sections.

Trauma Some injuries can result in blood appearing in your urine. For example, a fall astride the frame of your bike might damage your urethra. And some oddballs have been known to stick weird and wonderful things up there too. The kidneys can also be bruised or damaged – for example, by a kick or punch to the loin (the area each side of your lower back between the lowest part of your ribs and the highest part of your pelvis).

Treatment If you see blood in your wee after an injury, then go straight to casualty, as you may have done some serious damage.

Cancer of the kidney or bladder Bladder cancers usually show themselves by leaking blood into the urine – but bear in mind that they usually only happen in men over the age of 60. Kidney cancers are rarer, but can occur in a younger age group (under 40).

Treatment See your GP. If he's worried, he'll refer you to a urologist (waterworks specialist) for further tests.

Other medical rarities There are a number of unusual problems which can cause blood in your urine, including glomerulonephritis (inflamed kidneys), polycystic kidneys (swellings on the kidneys, which runs in families), and bleeding disorders (the blood is too thin and doesn't clot properly).

Treatment It's unlikely that you'll have any of these problems. Speak to your GP if you're concerned – he'll arrange any necessary tests.

Calf pain

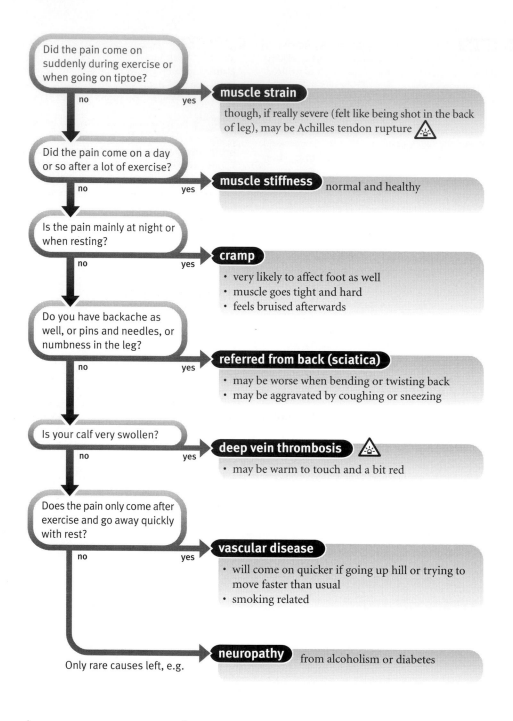

Did the pain come on suddenly during exercise or when going on tiptoe?

muscle strain

though, if really severe (felt like being shot in the back of leg), may be Achilles tendon rupture

Did the pain come on a day or so after a lot of exercise?

muscle stiffness normal and healthy

Is the pain mainly at night or when resting?

cramp

- very likely to affect foot as well
- muscle goes tight and hard
- feels bruised afterwards

Do you have backache as well, or pins and needles, or numbness in the leg?

referred from back (sciatica)

- may be worse when bending or twisting back
- may be aggravated by coughing or sneezing

Is your calf very swollen?

deep vein thrombosis

- may be warm to touch and a bit red

Does the pain only come after exercise and go away quickly with rest?

vascular disease

- will come on quicker if going up hill or trying to move faster than usual
- smoking related

Only rare causes left, e.g.

neuropathy from alcoholism or diabetes

Remember: ⚠ means see your GP sharpish; ⚠ means an urgent hospital job

Calf pain

Muscle strain If you overstretch a muscle, some of the individual strands which make up the muscle can tear, causing a sudden pain.

Treatment For a bad strain, you may need to rest the calf for a few days and use ice packs and painkillers (anti-inflammatory tablets such as ibuprofen – available from the chemist – can be particularly useful). Once the strain has healed, you will need to be careful with your normal sporting activities – if you do too much too soon, it'll flare up again. Remember warm-ups and stretching, as described below. A mild strain will get better within a few days and needs no special treatment, a more severe one may take six to eight weeks to heal.

Muscle stiffness (unaccustomed exercise) Muscles which haven't been used for a while can swell and become sore after a bout of exercise.

Treatment The pain will sort itself out after a day or two. The most you'll need is a simple painkiller like paracetamol. To prevent it happening in the future, improve your level of fitness, building up your exercise gradually, and doing a gentle warm-up and stretching routine before you really get going.

Cramp The calf muscles can go into spasm, causing severe pain at the time and leaving the area with a bruised feeling for a day or two afterwards. It's usually caused by being unfit or overdoing the exercise.

Treatment An attack of cramp can be cured simply by stretching the calf muscle – straighten the affected leg and, with your hand, pull your foot up towards you. Preventive measures include drinking enough fluids (especially before and after exercise), keeping reasonably fit, and warming up before any exertion. Stretching the calf muscles before exercise and bedtime will also prevent cramp – stretch the muscle a few times, just as you would for an attack of cramp. If all else fails and it's becoming a real problem, speak to your GP – sometimes tablets can help.

Referred from back Referred pain is pain which comes from one area but is felt in another. Back trouble – especially 'sciatica' – can cause pain in the calf.

Treatment See 'Back pain' section (p. 23).

Achilles tendon tear The Achilles tendon is the thick cord you can feel which attaches the lower end of your calf to your heel. A sudden stretch, especially going on tiptoe, can tear the tendon.

Treatment A suspected Achilles tendon tear needs urgent attention – go to casualty.

Deep vein thrombosis The arteries take blood to the leg muscles; the veins drain it back again. A clot – a liver-like lump – can form in one of these large veins. It's rare in men, and when it does occur, it's usually linked to a combination of smoking and being immobile – for example, being in a plaster because of a broken leg.

Treatment Check it urgently with your GP: if he thinks you have a thrombosis it'll mean a trip to the hospital for blood-thinning tablets to dissolve the clot.

Vascular disease Blood vessels (arteries) carry blood into the legs to supply the muscles with oxygen. If the arteries get furred up, the muscles can suffer from a lack of blood, especially during exercise. They complain by causing pain. This is rare in young men, but one type – Buerger's disease – can very occasionally affect male smokers under the age of 45.

Treatment Stop smoking, keep exercising, and take half a soluble aspirin a day – all of these measures help to unblock the arteries. But it's worth seeing your GP, as you will need to see a specialist for further tests and treatment.

Neuropathy This is a disease of the nerves supplying sensation to the legs. It can be caused by a whole variety of problems, most of which are pretty rare. The two commonest culprits in young men are diabetes and excessive boozing: the high blood sugar and the alcohol, respectively, poison the nerves.

Treatment If alcohol is the cause, you've obviously got to stop, as you have a serious problem and are probably an alcoholic. If you're having trouble stopping, or you think there might be some other cause – or you're known to be diabetic and you're wondering if you've developed neuropathy – see your GP.

Chest pain

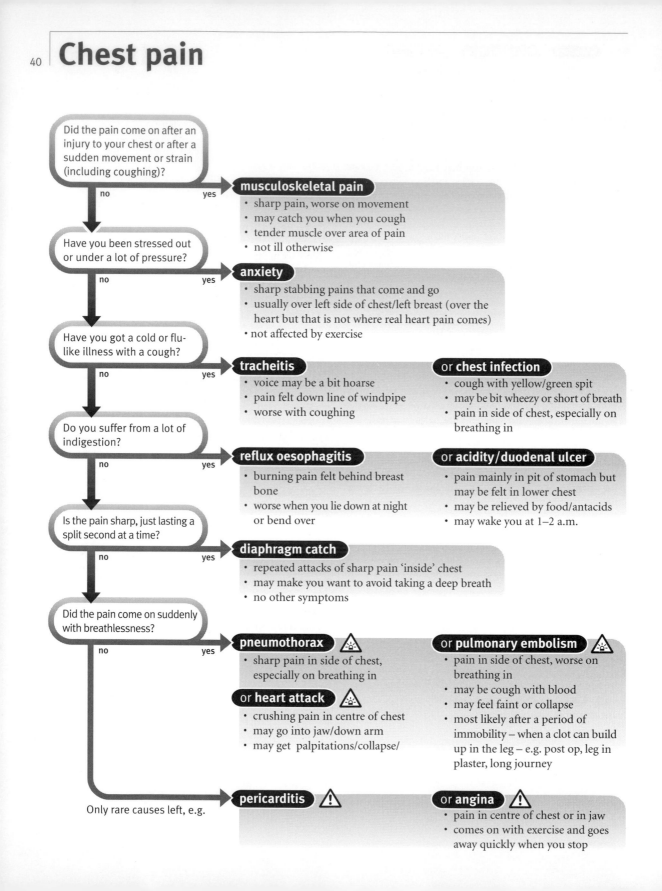

Did the pain come on after an injury to your chest or after a sudden movement or strain (including coughing)?

no / yes

musculoskeletal pain
- sharp pain, worse on movement
- may catch you when you cough
- tender muscle over area of pain
- not ill otherwise

Have you been stressed out or under a lot of pressure?

no / yes

anxiety
- sharp stabbing pains that come and go
- usually over left side of chest/left breast (over the heart but that is not where real heart pain comes)
- not affected by exercise

Have you got a cold or flu-like illness with a cough?

no / yes

tracheitis
- voice may be a bit hoarse
- pain felt down line of windpipe
- worse with coughing

or chest infection
- cough with yellow/green spit
- may be bit wheezy or short of breath
- pain in side of chest, especially on breathing in

Do you suffer from a lot of indigestion?

no / yes

reflux oesophagitis
- burning pain felt behind breast bone
- worse when you lie down at night or bend over

or acidity/duodenal ulcer
- pain mainly in pit of stomach but may be felt in lower chest
- may be relieved by food/antacids
- may wake you at 1–2 a.m.

Is the pain sharp, just lasting a split second at a time?

no / yes

diaphragm catch
- repeated attacks of sharp pain 'inside' chest
- may make you want to avoid taking a deep breath
- no other symptoms

Did the pain come on suddenly with breathlessness?

no / yes

pneumothorax
- sharp pain in side of chest, especially on breathing in

or heart attack
- crushing pain in centre of chest
- may go into jaw/down arm
- may get palpitations/collapse/

or pulmonary embolism
- pain in side of chest, worse on breathing in
- may be cough with blood
- may feel faint or collapse
- most likely after a period of immobility – when a clot can build up in the leg – e.g. post op, leg in plaster, long journey

Only rare causes left, e.g.

pericarditis

or angina
- pain in centre of chest or in jaw
- comes on with exercise and goes away quickly when you stop

Chest pain

Musculoskeletal pain The muscle and bone which make up the rib cage can be inflamed by a muscle strain, a knock, or a virus.

Treatment This will settle down on its own, but can take up to a few weeks because the rib cage is very sensitive and is in constant 'use' (expanding and contracting with every breath you take). Painkillers or anti-inflammatories (such as ibuprofen) from the chemist will help, as will heat treatment (like a heat lamp or a hot water bottle).

Anxiety Feeling uptight tenses the muscles in the rib cage, which can cause various types of pains. If you're already anxious and you start getting chest pains, you're likely to worry that you've got something serious wrong, such as heart trouble. This creates more anxiety and worsening pains, and so a vicious cycle develops.

Treatment The key thing is to accept there's nothing seriously wrong, as this will help you relax, easing the muscle tension. If you have trouble convincing yourself, discuss the situation with your GP. Also, try to sort out whatever is making you uptight in the first place; relaxation exercises and physical exercise will help too. For further details, see the 'Feeling tense' section (p. 59).

Tracheitis If you have a cold or the flu, the germ can go down your windpipe (the 'trachea'), causing tracheitis.

Treatment Antibiotics don't help. It'll go away on its own in a few days – in the meantime, try painkillers and steam inhalations, and avoid cigarette smoke.

Reflux oesophagitis This is explained, and the treatment outlined, in the 'Indigestion' section (p. 71). If the acid makes the gullet very sore, it can cause a pain felt in the chest.

Diaphragm catch The diaphragm is the internal sheet of muscle separating your chest from your guts. Diaphragm catch is thought to be an irritation of this muscle, although no one knows what causes it – but it's definitely harmless.

Treatment As the cause isn't known, there's nothing that you can really do to prevent it. It comes on and disappears so quickly it's not even worth taking a painkiller, as the pain will go long before any tablet has a chance to work. So just try to ignore it.

Acidity/duodenal ulcer This is explained, and the treatment discussed, in the 'Abdominal pain – recurrent' section (p. 15). Sometimes the pain is felt in the chest rather than the belly.

Chest infection A severe type of chest infection – pneumonia – can cause 'pleurisy'. This is explained further in the 'Cough' section (p. 43).

Angina or heart attack If the blood vessels which feed your heart get furred up, blood can have trouble getting through. As a result, the heart muscle gets starved of oxygen and complains by producing a tight pain across the chest, particularly when you're exerting yourself – this is 'angina'. It's pretty unlikely in the under 35s. If a blood vessel blocks totally, then the bit of heart muscle it supplies dies – this causes a sudden and severe pain across the chest (a heart attack or 'myocardial infarction'). Any bloke can suffer from heart trouble, especially as he gets older, but it's more likely if you smoke, have heart disease in the family, are overweight, eat a lousy diet, have a high cholesterol level (a type of fat in the blood), have high blood pressure, or do little exercise – and particularly if you have any combination of these.

Treatment If you think you're getting angina, you must see your GP. He'll probably start you on some medication; he'll also refer you to a heart specialist for further tests to confirm that this is the problem and to see if you need any other types of treatment. It's very important to sort out your lifestyle: your GP will give you advice about diet, weight loss, and exercise, and you'll need to pack up the fags. If you think you might be having a heart attack, don't mess about – call an ambulance straight away. The hospital doctors can give you treatment to ease the pain and protect your heart, but this has to be done as soon as possible. And while you're waiting for the paramedics, chew an aspirin, because this thins the blood and helps unblock the blood vessels.

Pericarditis This is an inflammation of the lining of the heart, which is usually caused by a virus.

Treatment You'll need to see your GP, who may well send you to hospital if he thinks you've got pericarditis.

Pneumothorax and pulmonary embolism These are explained in the 'Shortness of breath' (p. 123) and 'Blood in spit' (p. 35) sections.

Cough

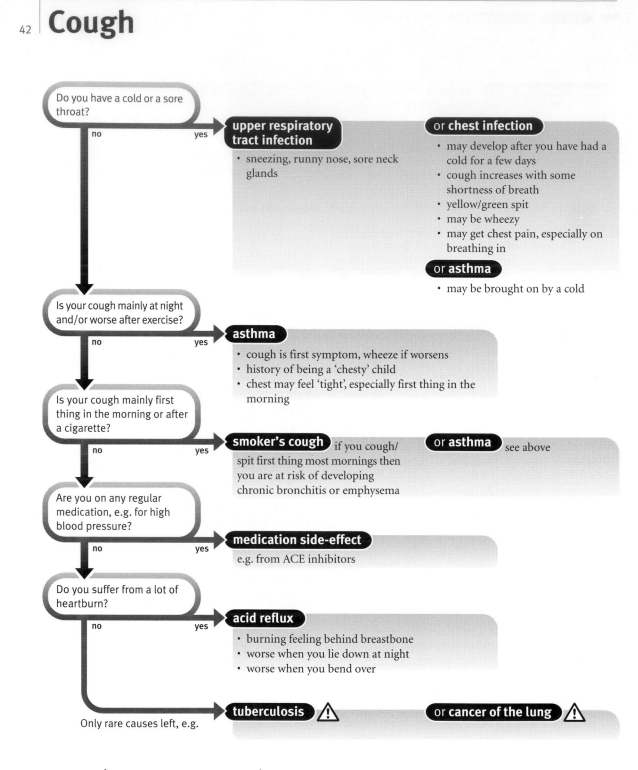

Do you have a cold or a sore throat?
no   yes

upper respiratory tract infection
- sneezing, runny nose, sore neck glands

or chest infection
- may develop after you have had a cold for a few days
- cough increases with some shortness of breath
- yellow/green spit
- may be wheezy
- may get chest pain, especially on breathing in

or asthma
- may be brought on by a cold

Is your cough mainly at night and/or worse after exercise?
no   yes

asthma
- cough is first symptom, wheeze if worsens
- history of being a 'chesty' child
- chest may feel 'tight', especially first thing in the morning

Is your cough mainly first thing in the morning or after a cigarette?
no   yes

smoker's cough if you cough/spit first thing most mornings then you are at risk of developing chronic bronchitis or emphysema

or asthma see above

Are you on any regular medication, e.g. for high blood pressure?
no   yes

medication side-effect
e.g. from ACE inhibitors

Do you suffer from a lot of heartburn?
no   yes

acid reflux
- burning feeling behind breastbone
- worse when you lie down at night
- worse when you bend over

Only rare causes left, e.g.

tuberculosis ⚠

or cancer of the lung ⚠

Remember: ⚠ means see your GP sharpish; ⚠ means an urgent hospital job

NB In every case, smoking will aggravate the problem and may, if continued, make it more likely to come back again in the future. So we'll say it only once to avoid repetition: cut down – or better still, stop – smoking. More detail is provided in the 'Shortness of breath' section (p. 123).

Upper respiratory tract infection The upper respiratory tract includes the ear, nose, throat, and windpipe. Infections are usually caused by viruses, the commonest resulting in the humble cold.

Treatment Paracetamol and a high fluid intake will ease the aches and pains and sore throat. Inhaling steam from a bowl of hot water, with a towel over your head (add menthol if you like) and propping yourself up at night will help the cough, whereas cough mixtures probably don't achieve a lot. The cough does have a purpose – it's the body's way of getting the germ out of your windpipe – so it's not surprising that it can take a week or two to go. And if the cold leaves you with lots of catarrh, this can drip down the back of the throat, especially at night, making the cough drag on. Again, inhalations may help. Don't bother your GP with this problem, though, because there's really nothing to do other than give it time to settle.

Chest infection There are various types, the most likely being bronchitis. This is a complication of an upper respiratory tract infection (see above) in which the germ gets into the lungs. But if you're really ill, you might have pneumonia – a severe form of chest infection which can spread to the lining of the lung causing 'pleurisy'. This is more likely to be a complication of flu or chickenpox rather than a simple cold.

Treatment If your cough is showing no signs of settling after a few days with the treatment described for upper respiratory tract infection, or if you feel really rough or are having any trouble breathing, then it's worth seeing your GP – you may need antibiotics to clear the germ. And if it turns out you have pneumonia, you might even need to be admitted to hospital.

Smoker's cough Cigarette smoke irritates the lungs, causing a cough. It also makes the lungs produce more protective mucus, which builds up as catarrh – this can only be shifted by coughing, and is often noticed more first thing in the morning. Remember that you don't necessarily have to be a smoker to develop a smoker's cough – breathing in other people's smoke (passive smoking) can cause it too.

Treatment See the 'Smoking' part of the 'Shortness of breath' section (p. 123).

Asthma If the small airways in the lung narrow at times and clog up with phlegm, the result is a cough, wheezing, and shortness of breath. This is asthma. The exact cause is unknown, but it can run in families, is linked to hay fever and eczema, and can be triggered by certain things, such as colds, pollen, changes in air temperature, stress, and exercise.

Treatment See your GP. You're likely to be prescribed treatment in the form of inhalers, which should sort out the problem, provided you use them as directed. There's not much you can do to prevent attacks unless there's obviously something that brings it on and which you can avoid (such as an allergy to cats). It's a sensible idea to keep in shape – swimming is thought to be particularly good exercise for asthmatics. If you're coughing a lot and are really tight-chested – or you're known to have asthma and you think your coughing is caused by a bad attack – then see your GP urgently as you may need some other treatment such as steroid tablets.

Medication side-effect One group of treatments often prescribed for blood pressure problems in young men – 'ACE inhibitors' – have cough as their main side-effect.

Treatment Discuss the situation with your GP. You'll either need to put up with the cough – if it isn't too troublesome – or be switched to a different type of blood pressure pill.

Acid reflux If the valve at the top of your stomach doesn't work properly, the acid in your stomach can leak up into your gullet – this is acid reflux. When you lie down, it can spill right up into the throat, causing spasms of coughing.

Treatment Lose weight if you're fat, don't eat too late at night, and try an antacid from the chemist. Also, raise the head of your bed a couple of inches with blocks – gravity will then keep the acid in your stomach when you're asleep.

Rare medical causes There is a whole heap of very unusual causes. Cancer is rare in the under 45s, and incredibly unlikely in non-smokers. Other possibilities include TB and rare lung diseases. You're unlikely to need to worry about any of these.

Treatment See your GP. If he's concerned, he'll arrange the necessary tests.

Deafness

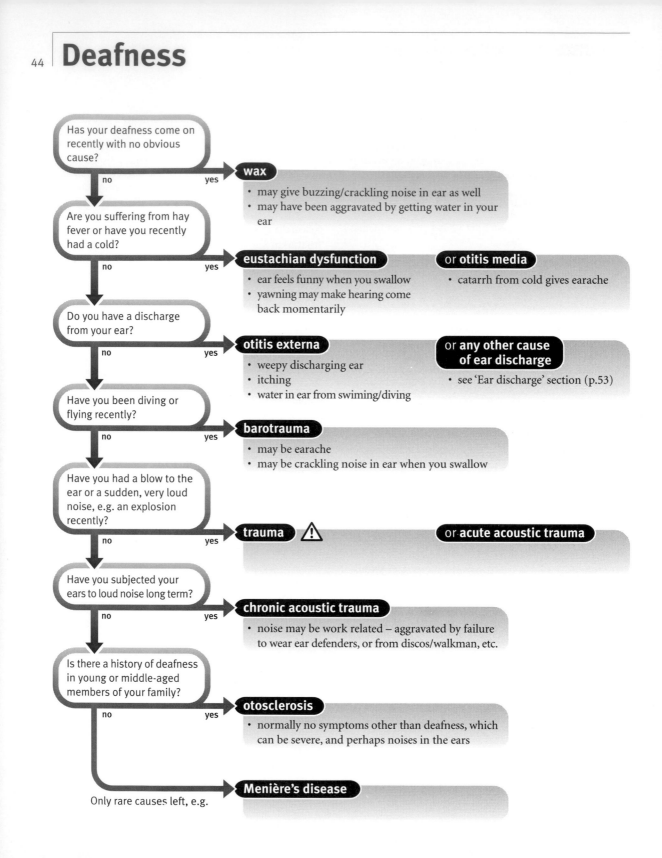

Has your deafness come on recently with no obvious cause?

no / yes

wax
- may give buzzing/crackling noise in ear as well
- may have been aggravated by getting water in your ear

Are you suffering from hay fever or have you recently had a cold?

no / yes

eustachian dysfunction
- ear feels funny when you swallow
- yawning may make hearing come back momentarily

or otitis media
- catarrh from cold gives earache

Do you have a discharge from your ear?

no / yes

otitis externa
- weepy discharging ear
- itching
- water in ear from swiming/diving

or any other cause of ear discharge
- see 'Ear discharge' section (p.53)

Have you been diving or flying recently?

no / yes

barotrauma
- may be earache
- may be crackling noise in ear when you swallow

Have you had a blow to the ear or a sudden, very loud noise, e.g. an explosion recently?

no / yes

trauma ⚠

or acute acoustic trauma

Have you subjected your ears to loud noise long term?

no / yes

chronic acoustic trauma
- noise may be work related – aggravated by failure to wear ear defenders, or from discos/walkman, etc.

Is there a history of deafness in young or middle-aged members of your family?

no / yes

otosclerosis
- normally no symptoms other than deafness, which can be severe, and perhaps noises in the ears

Only rare causes left, e.g.

Menière's disease

Ear wax The ear canal (the tube you can put your little finger into and which leads to your ear drum) produces wax. This is quite normal, but if a lot of wax builds up – or it becomes wedged down inside the canal because you've been ramming cotton buds in your ear – it can block the ear canal completely, causing deafness.

Treatment Don't try to gouge the wax out yourself. Cotton buds will just push it down further and harden it, making it more difficult to shift. Instead, soften the wax for a couple of days using ear drops from the chemist. This may solve the problem. If it doesn't, see your GP or practice nurse, who will probably syringe the wax out for you.

Eustachian tube dysfunction The eustachian tube is the internal tube which connects the inner part of the ear to the back of the throat. Its job is to equalize pressure changes and drain catarrh from the ear. When it gets blocked – most commonly because of a cold or hay fever – it doesn't work properly (eustachian tube dysfunction), causing a build-up of catarrh which results in deafness.

Treatment Usually, the problem sorts itself out on its own within a few days. Inhaling steam from a bowl of hot water, with some added menthol, may help by shifting some of the catarrh. If it drags on for a while, a technique called the Valsalva manoeuvre is worth trying. The trick is to build up air pressure in your mouth and throat – this can open up the eustachian tube. The easiest way to do this is to simply blow up a balloon. You may need to keep trying this for some days – eventually, the ear should start to crackle or pop, and the deafness will clear. If the cause might be hay fever, try one of the over-the-counter anti-hay fever nose sprays, as this is likely to solve the problem.

Otitis media This is explained in the 'Earache' section (p. 51). The infection inflames the drum, causing deafness.

Treatment See the 'Earache' section (p. 51). The deafness is usually the last symptom to settle – it may take a few weeks before your hearing seems completely normal again.

Any cause of ear discharge Various problems – particularly infections – can cause a discharge from the ear (see the 'Ear discharge' section, p. 53). If the discharge blocks the ear canal, then your hearing is bound to be affected.

Treatment See the 'Ear discharge' section (p. 53).

Barotrauma This is the term used to describe problems caused by outside pressure changes affecting the ear. The most common causes are air travel and scuba diving – the deafness results from a build-up of fluid deep inside the ear and is especially likely if these activities are done when you have a cold.

Treatment The problem will correct itself, but it can take many weeks. The tricks described under eustachian tube dysfunction (above) may help.

Acoustic trauma This can be sudden or from long term damage and is explained in the section on 'Noises in the ear' (p. 93).

Treatment There is no magic cure. Discuss the situation with your GP if it is becoming a problem – he may refer you to an Ear, Nose, and Throat ('ENT') specialist to consider a hearing aid.

Otosclerosis The inside of the ear contains tiny bones which move to amplify the sound. These bones can sometimes stiffen up and not move as they should, causing deafness which slowly gets worse – this is otosclerosis. This problem can run in families.

Treatment You will need to see an ENT specialist to confirm this diagnosis. If necessary, it can be treated with surgery.

Trauma This is explained, and the treatment outlined, in the 'Earache' section (p. 51).

Menière's disease This is a disease caused by an increase in the pressure of the fluid which circulates in the deepest, most complex parts of the ear. This high pressure affects the hearing and balance apparatus, resulting in deafness, dizziness, and ringing in the ears. Quite why it should happen remains unclear.

Treatment See your GP – it's likely that you'll be referred to an ENT specialist to be checked out.

Other rare causes These include small print diseases such as unusual viruses, types of stroke, and growths on the nerve of the ear.

Treatment Discuss the problem with your GP, who will arrange any necessary tests or hospital appointments.

Diarrhoea

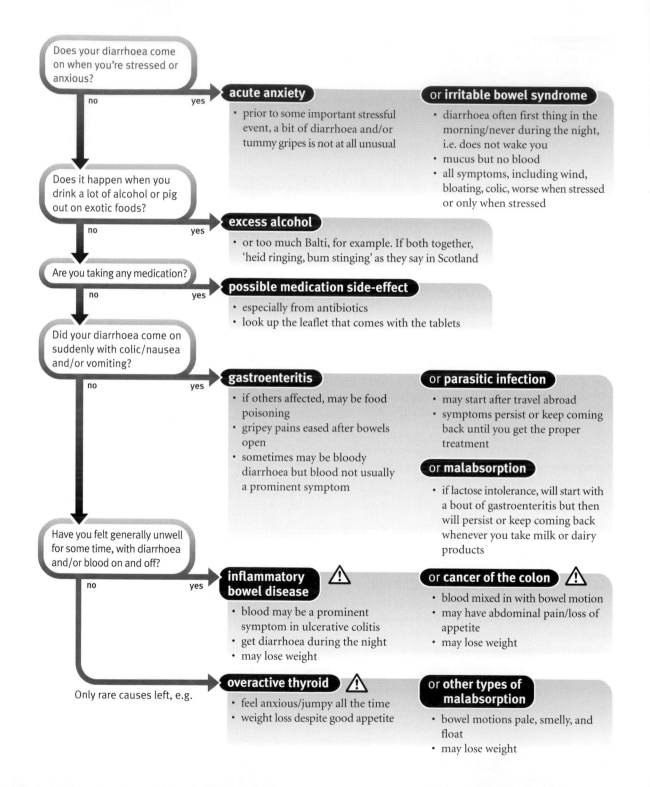

Does your diarrhoea come on when you're stressed or anxious?

no / yes

acute anxiety
- prior to some important stressful event, a bit of diarrhoea and/or tummy gripes is not at all unusual

or irritable bowel syndrome
- diarrhoea often first thing in the morning/never during the night, i.e. does not wake you
- mucus but no blood
- all symptoms, including wind, bloating, colic, worse when stressed or only when stressed

Does it happen when you drink a lot of alcohol or pig out on exotic foods?

no / yes

excess alcohol
- or too much Balti, for example. If both together, 'heid ringing, bum stinging' as they say in Scotland

Are you taking any medication?

no / yes

possible medication side-effect
- especially from antibiotics
- look up the leaflet that comes with the tablets

Did your diarrhoea come on suddenly with colic/nausea and/or vomiting?

no / yes

gastroenteritis
- if others affected, may be food poisoning
- gripey pains eased after bowels open
- sometimes may be bloody diarrhoea but blood not usually a prominent symptom

or parasitic infection
- may start after travel abroad
- symptoms persist or keep coming back until you get the proper treatment

or malabsorption
- if lactose intolerance, will start with a bout of gastroenteritis but then will persist or keep coming back whenever you take milk or dairy products

Have you felt generally unwell for some time, with diarrhoea and/or blood on and off?

no / yes

inflammatory bowel disease ⚠
- blood may be a prominent symptom in ulcerative colitis
- get diarrhoea during the night
- may lose weight

or cancer of the colon ⚠
- blood mixed in with bowel motion
- may have abdominal pain/loss of appetite
- may lose weight

Only rare causes left, e.g.

overactive thyroid ⚠
- feel anxious/jumpy all the time
- weight loss despite good appetite

or other types of malabsorption
- bowel motions pale, smelly, and float
- may lose weight

Acute anxiety Important life events like exams, driving tests, weddings, court appearances, and so on can make your bowel overactive – especially first thing in the morning when you get up.

Treatment This is totally normal, so no treatment is needed.

Excess alcohol Drinking too much – especially binge drinking – often results in diarrhoea. The sheer volume of fluid may be the cause, or it might be that you have mild irritable bowel syndrome, which is aggravated by alcohol. On the other hand, it might have something to do with the fact that your alcohol intake is closely linked to other gut irritants such as vindaloos.

Treatment Cut down on the booze – and avoid binges.

Gastroenteritis A germ in the bowel, usually through something you've eaten – hence the term 'food poisoning'.

Treatment This is covered in the 'Abdominal pain-one off' section (p. 13).

Irritable bowel syndrome (IBS) The bowel is simply a long muscular tube. When 'irritable', it squeezes too much, too little, or in an uncoordinated way, resulting in the typical symptoms of IBS.

Treatment Most of the treatment is covered in the 'Abdominal pain – recurrent' section (p. 15). When diarrhoea is the main symptom, an over-the-counter medicine, such as loperamide, may help, although medicines like this are probably best kept to a minimum. Cutting down your fibre intake may also help – but could cause problems too if you also get constipated at times with your IBS.

Medication side-effect Just about any medication – prescribed or bought over-the-counter – can cause diarrhoea. The worst culprits are probably antibiotics and anti-inflammatory drugs like ibuprofen.

Treatment Try to grin and bear it if the treatment is just a short course, such as a few days of antibiotics for an infection. If that seems impossible, seek an alternative medicine: your pharmacist or GP will be able to help you. If the diarrhoea seems to be a side-effect of long-term medication prescribed by your doctor, you'll need to discuss the situation with him. You may be advised to try without the treatment, or you might be prescribed something else instead.

Malabsorption Some diseases of the gut stop your food being broken down (i.e. digested) or taken into the body (i.e. absorbed) properly. This leads to diarrhoea, and is known as malabsorption. Two of the commonest causes are coeliac disease, in which you cannot absorb gluten (found in wheat, rye, barley, and oats), and lactose intolerance, in which you cannot tolerate lactose (a sugar found in milk).

Treatment You will need to see your GP. He'll look into it either by arranging special tests or by sending you to a dietitian who, by cutting out certain items in your diet, will be able to work out what the precise problem is. The dietitian is obviously helpful in treatment too, as the cure often lies in knowing which foods to avoid. Other types of malabsorption may need specialist treatment.

Parasitic infections Some unusual infections of the gut are caused by parasites (organisms which live off other organisms). These microscopic creatures live in the wall of the bowel, causing, amongst other symptoms, diarrhoea. They are usually – but not always – picked up from travel abroad.

Treatment If you think you may have this type of problem, see your GP. You'll need tests and, if they confirm the diagnosis, a course of antibiotics.

Inflammatory bowel disease Crohn's disease and ulcerative colitis are the 'inflammatory bowel diseases' – illnesses which inflame the lining of the gut, causing diarrhoea which may be bloody, often with other symptoms like weight loss. The precise cause remains a mystery.

Treatment See your GP. He will arrange tests, which will usually include seeing a gut specialist in hospital. Your treatment will depend on the type of disease you have, and its pattern, and may involve tablets – sometimes lifelong – and enemas (liquids squirted up into the bottom).

Overactive thyroid The thyroid gland sits in the middle of the front of the neck, around the Adam's apple. It produces thyroid hormone, which controls the body's activity. If too much is produced – 'hyperthyroidism' – one of the effects is persistent diarrhoea.

Treatment This is covered in the 'Excess sweating' section (p. 55).

Colon cancer The colon is the large bowel – the last part of your gut which ends up at the rectum and anus (back passage). Colon cancer is rare in the under 40s. However, there is some increase in risk if you have had polyps (small benign growths) of the colon – or they run in your family – or you've had severe ulcerative colitis for years.

Treatment See your GP, who will arrange the necessary tests and an appointment with a specialist.

Dizziness

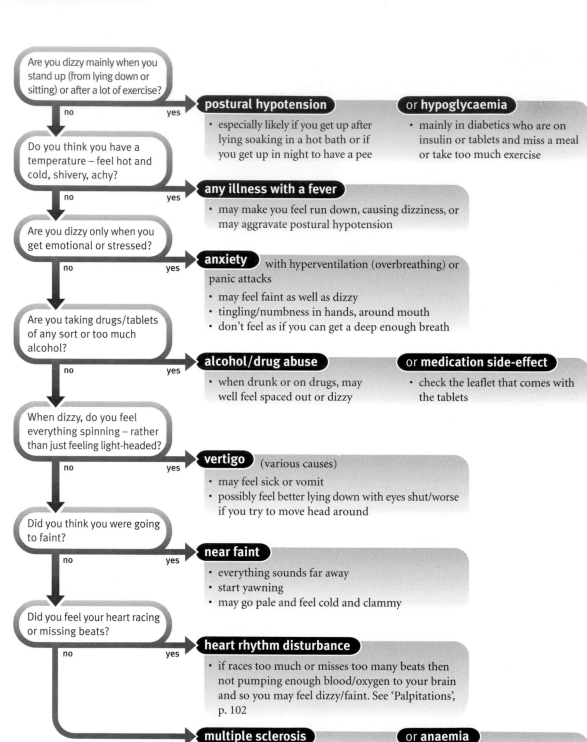

Are you dizzy mainly when you stand up (from lying down or sitting) or after a lot of exercise?

yes → **postural hypotension**
- especially likely if you get up after lying soaking in a hot bath or if you get up in night to have a pee

or hypoglycaemia
- mainly in diabetics who are on insulin or tablets and miss a meal or take too much exercise

no ↓

Do you think you have a temperature – feel hot and cold, shivery, achy?

yes → **any illness with a fever**
- may make you feel run down, causing dizziness, or may aggravate postural hypotension

no ↓

Are you dizzy only when you get emotional or stressed?

yes → **anxiety** with hyperventilation (overbreathing) or panic attacks
- may feel faint as well as dizzy
- tingling/numbness in hands, around mouth
- don't feel as if you can get a deep enough breath

no ↓

Are you taking drugs/tablets of any sort or too much alcohol?

yes → **alcohol/drug abuse**
- when drunk or on drugs, may well feel spaced out or dizzy

or medication side-effect
- check the leaflet that comes with the tablets

no ↓

When dizzy, do you feel everything spinning – rather than just feeling light-headed?

yes → **vertigo** (various causes)
- may feel sick or vomit
- possibly feel better lying down with eyes shut/worse if you try to move head around

no ↓

Did you think you were going to faint?

yes → **near faint**
- everything sounds far away
- start yawning
- may go pale and feel cold and clammy

no ↓

Did you feel your heart racing or missing beats?

yes → **heart rhythm disturbance**
- if races too much or misses too many beats then not pumping enough blood/oxygen to your brain and so you may feel dizzy/faint. See 'Palpitations', p. 102

no ↓

multiple sclerosis **or anaemia**

Only rare causes left, e.g.

Postural hypotension If you stand up suddenly, your blood pressure can drop. Momentarily, not enough blood gets through to the brain, which is starved of oxygen for a few seconds. The result is light-headedness, which quickly passes off. A typical example is when you leap out of a hot bath to answer the 'phone.

Treatment This type of dizziness is almost always normal, although it can be made worse by some prescribed treatments (such as blood pressure pills and antidepressants). Talk to your GP if you think that your treatment is causing you a problem.

Any illness with a high temperature Feeling a bit light-headed – especially on standing – is a common symptom whenever you've got a virus or some other infection (e.g. flu, a tummy bug, tonsillitis, or a chest infection).

Treatment The dizziness itself doesn't need treatment as it's simply part of the overall grotty feeling. Use your main symptom (such as cough and sore throat) to guide you to the right section of this book.

Anxiety Being uptight can make you feel dizzy, especially if it leads to hyperventilation or panic attacks. See the 'Feeling tense' (p. 59) or 'Shortness of breath' (p. 123) sections for further details and advice about treatment.

Alcohol and drug abuse It's hardly surprising that you'll feel dizzy when the aim is to get out of your head.

Treatment The dizziness itself isn't harmful, unless of course you keel over and injure yourself. But drug and alcohol abuse obviously can be. If you think you have a problem and you want help, see your GP or contact the local drug or alcohol unit.

Vertigo This is the medical word to describe an unpleasant 'head spinning' feeling (like when you've just stepped off a carousel). It's caused by something going wrong with your balance mechanism, and there are lots of different causes. In blokes, the most common are viral labyrinthitis (a germ affecting the ear, usually with a cold) and benign positional vertigo (vertigo which keeps coming on whenever you turn your head in certain positions). Drinking a few too many lagers can have a very similar effect.

Treatment This depends on the cause, so you'll need to speak to your GP. The viral type goes away on its own, usually after a few days. Benign positional vertigo may need the help of an Ear, Nose, and Throat ('ENT') specialist. And remember not to drive until you can turn your head without the world spinning round.

Near faint A near faint is simply a faint that you just about manage to prevent – see the 'Loss of consciousness' section for more details.

Medication side-effect Some prescribed treatments can cause light-headedness. They can also lead to postural hypotension (see above).

Treatment Take a look at the leaflet in the pack. If it mentions dizziness, have a word with your GP – he may be able to stop the treatment or prescribe something else instead.

Hypoglycaemia This means a low blood sugar level. The sugar in your blood fuels the brain – so if the levels drop, maybe because you've missed a meal or you've done an unusual amount of exercise, you tend to feel a bit light-headed. This is particularly common in diabetics on treatment (the pills or injections lower the blood sugar).

Treatment Eat regularly and, in particular, don't skip breakfast. If you're a diabetic, check out the 'Hypoglycaemia' part of the 'Loss of consciousness' section (p. 81).

Heart rhythm disturbance If your heart beats too slowly, too quickly, or erratically, it may not pump enough blood through to the brain, causing dizziness – see the 'Palpitations' section, p. 103 (especially the 'Supraventricular tachycardia' part) for more details.

Rare medical problem A whole load of small print problems (including anaemia, multiple sclerosis, kidney failure, and heart valve problems) can cause dizziness, but you're highly unlikely to have any of them – and they tend to cause lots of other symptoms which give the game away.

Treatment If you think you might be suffering one of these rarities, you're probably wrong, but have a word with your GP.

Earache

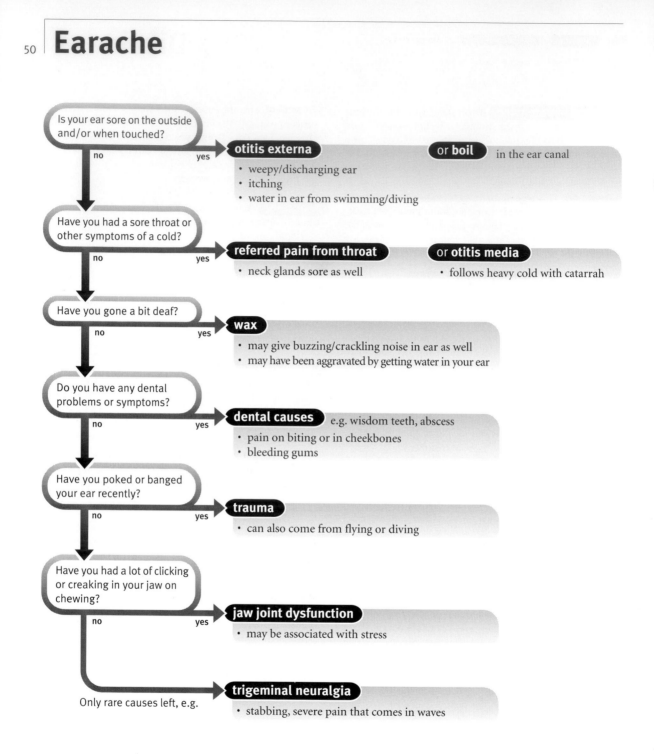

Is your ear sore on the outside and/or when touched?

no — yes →

otitis externa   or **boil** in the ear canal
- weepy/discharging ear
- itching
- water in ear from swimming/diving

Have you had a sore throat or other symptoms of a cold?

no — yes →

referred pain from throat   or **otitis media**
- neck glands sore as well   • follows heavy cold with catarrah

Have you gone a bit deaf?

no — yes →

wax
- may give buzzing/crackling noise in ear as well
- may have been aggravated by getting water in your ear

Do you have any dental problems or symptoms?

no — yes →

dental causes e.g. wisdom teeth, abscess
- pain on biting or in cheekbones
- bleeding gums

Have you poked or banged your ear recently?

no — yes →

trauma
- can also come from flying or diving

Have you had a lot of clicking or creaking in your jaw on chewing?

no — yes →

jaw joint dysfunction
- may be associated with stress

Only rare causes left, e.g.

trigeminal neuralgia
- stabbing, severe pain that comes in waves

Earache

Otitis externa An infection of the outer ear canal – the bit you can get your finger into.

Treatment If you keep water out of your ears and stop prodding about with cotton buds, then it may settle down on its own. Ban buds and water anyway in the long run to stop repeated attacks: the ear canal can clean itself without your help, and waterlogging can be avoided by using ear plugs (e.g. cotton wool dipped in vaseline) when washing your hair or swimming. For a bad attack, you'll need drops or a spray from your GP. And if you get eczema of the ear canal, hydrocortisone 1% cream from the chemist may help.

Boil This is just like a boil anywhere else – an infection of the skin which can develop into a pus-filled lump. Except that, being in the confined space of the ear canal, it hurts like stink.

Treatment Painkillers and cross your fingers – it's likely to go by itself in a few days, but, if it's getting worse, your GP may prescribe antibiotics.

Wax Most people react to wax by attacking their ears with cotton buds. This makes matters worse, as the wax simply gets wedged further in so that it presses on the ear drum, causing pain.

Treatment First, throw those buds away. Next, use drops from the chemist to soften the wax. This may solve the problem, but, if it just makes you deafer, see the practice nurse who will syringe it for you.

Otitis media An infection of the eardrum, usually with a cold. It's the commonest cause of earache in children.

Treatment Try some painkillers from the chemist for 24 hours. If it's showing no signs of improving, contact your GP, as you may need antibiotics.

Referred pain Problems in a variety of other areas can 'send' the pain to the ear. For example, throat infections and wear and tear of the bones in the neck can result in pain which feels as though it comes from the ear.

Treatment Figure out where it's coming from, look up the appropriate section in this book and, hey presto, problem solved.

Dental causes All sorts of dental problems, such as wisdom tooth trouble or abscesses, can result in earache.

Treatment Bite the bullet and see a dentist.

Trauma Assaulting your ear runs the risk of causing damage – probably just a scrape to the canal, though you can knacker the eardrum if you're really determined. A loud noise or a smack to the side of the head (which includes a badly executed dive into a swimming pool) can also cause painful damage. Pressure changes – called 'barotrauma' – which you might feel when flying or scuba diving can also cause earache.

Treatment Sudden pain after trauma, especially with deafness, is not good news – you may have done some significant damage. See your doctor asap or go to casualty. The ache caused by barotrauma usually settles down quickly, although your hearing may feel a bit muffled for a week or two.

Jaw joint dysfunction A problem of the hinge joint between the jaw and the skull – there's one on each side, right next to each ear. If your bite is slightly out of line, or you grind your teeth out of habit or when tense, the joint can get inflamed and painful.

Treatment Use painkillers for a bad attack, but to get it cured you probably need to see your dentist.

Trigeminal neuralgia Neuralgia is a sharp pain coming from a nerve – in this case, the 'trigeminal', which supplies the sensation to the ear.

Treatment Wait and see. It'll probably fizzle out on its own after a while. If not, discuss the situation with your doctor.

Ear discharge

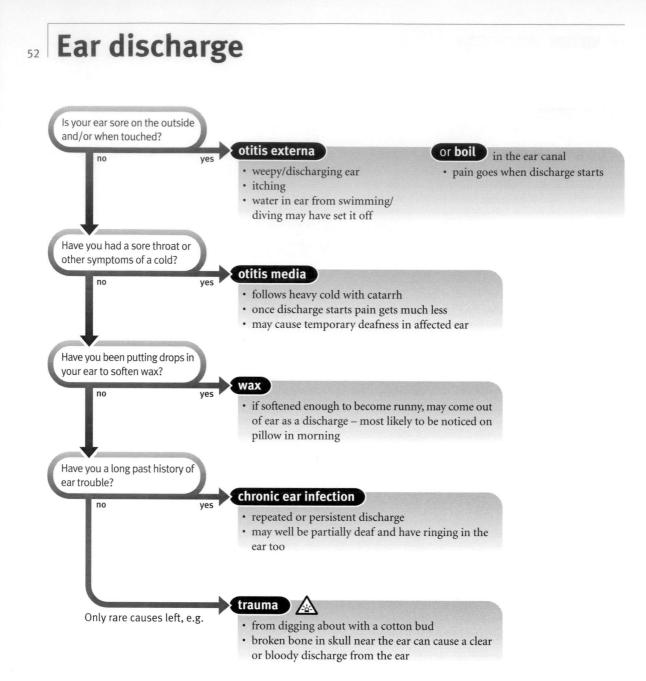

Is your ear sore on the outside and/or when touched?

no   yes

otitis externa
- weepy/discharging ear
- itching
- water in ear from swimming/ diving may have set it off

or **boil** in the ear canal
- pain goes when discharge starts

Have you had a sore throat or other symptoms of a cold?

no   yes

otitis media
- follows heavy cold with catarrh
- once discharge starts pain gets much less
- may cause temporary deafness in affected ear

Have you been putting drops in your ear to soften wax?

no   yes

wax
- if softened enough to become runny, may come out of ear as a discharge – most likely to be noticed on pillow in morning

Have you a long past history of ear trouble?

no   yes

chronic ear infection
- repeated or persistent discharge
- may well be partially deaf and have ringing in the ear too

Only rare causes left, e.g.

trauma
- from digging about with a cotton bud
- broken bone in skull near the ear can cause a clear or bloody discharge from the ear

Remember: ⚠ means see your GP sharpish; ⚠ means an urgent hospital job

Otitis externa This is explained, and its treatment outlined, in the 'Earache' section (p. 51).

Boil This is an infection which produces a lump full of pus. This can happen in the ear canal where, because of the confined space, it'll hurt like hell. If you just grit your teeth, or load yourself with painkillers, you'll find either that the boil just disappears, or it bursts, leaking a discharge out of your ear.

Treatment By the time the boil is discharging, it's curing itself. The pain usually eases as soon as the discharge starts. The muck should disappear after a couple of days – if it doesn't, get your GP to take a look.

Otitis media This is an infection of the eardrum, usually with a cold. Pus can build up under pressure behind the eardrum, causing pain and, sometimes, a hole in the drum, so the pus escapes in the form of an ear discharge.

Treatment As the discharge starts, the pain usually eases up, because the pressure on the eardrum is relieved. Unless the discharge and pain settle down quickly over a day or so, this type of infection requires antibiotics (in the form of medicine or drops) – so see your GP. The fact that your ear has discharged means that there must be a hole in your eardrum. This can take a few weeks to heal, so don't be surprised if your hearing seems dodgy for a while (and keep water out of your ears until everything seems back to normal). If the discharge keeps coming back, or your hearing isn't 100% again after a month, get your GP to take another look.

Wax It's normal to have wax in your ears. Some people seem to produce loads, others hardly any. If you have a build-up of wax, it can come out as a hard lump or as runny, brown goo. The latter is particularly likely if you've been using ear drops, maybe because the excess wax was making you deaf.

Treatment As wax is normal, it doesn't need treatment. Clean up any wax you can see, but avoid the temptation to attack your ear canal (the bit you can get your little finger into) with cotton buds – this simply wedges the wax back in and can damage your eardrum.

Chronic ear infection Sometimes, an infection like otitis media fails to clear or keeps coming back. This is known as a chronic ear infection (the chronic refers to the fact that it carries on a long time, not that it is more painful than other types of ear infection). It usually means that the eardrum still has a hole in it which won't heal, and it can result in a lot of damage to your hearing apparatus.

Treatment Get it checked out by your GP; if he can't sort it out, he'll refer you to an Ear, Nose, and Throat ('ENT') specialist.

Trauma The most likely type of trauma involves you digging around with a cotton bud. This can graze the ear canal, causing a slight bleed. But if you're really determined, you can damage the eardrum, in which case you'll get pain, blood, and a sudden problem with your hearing. Another, less likely, type of trauma is a serious head injury causing a broken bone in the skull near your ear. This can result in the ear losing a bloody or clear discharge.

Treatment If it's just a graze, don't worry about it – it'll heal itself. Just avoid cotton buds in future. If you think you've done more serious damage, seek medical help asap. And if you've fractured a bone in your skull – you won't be reading this, because you'll be in casualty.

Excess sweating

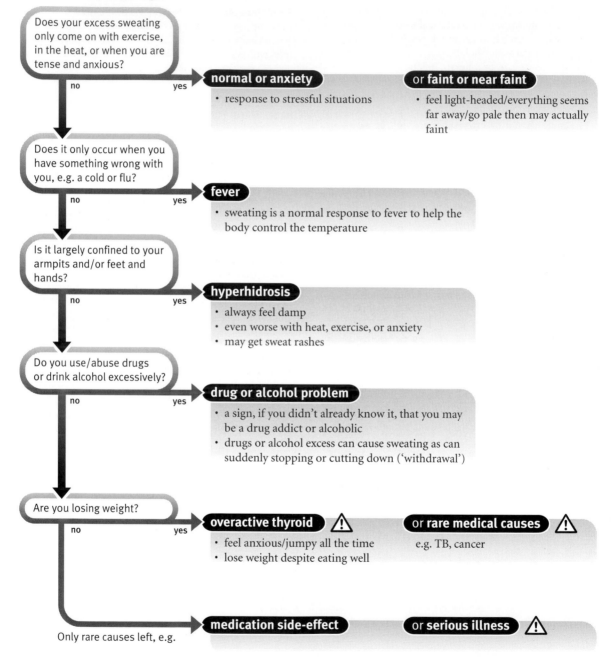

If you are a diabetic on treatment, excess sweating may be a sign you are going 'hypo' (hypoglycaemic) – if in doubt, take sugar.

Does your excess sweating only come on with exercise, in the heat, or when you are tense and anxious?
— no / yes →

normal or anxiety
- response to stressful situations

or faint or near faint
- feel light-headed/everything seems far away/go pale then may actually faint

Does it only occur when you have something wrong with you, e.g. a cold or flu?
— no / yes →

fever
- sweating is a normal response to fever to help the body control the temperature

Is it largely confined to your armpits and/or feet and hands?
— no / yes →

hyperhidrosis
- always feel damp
- even worse with heat, exercise, or anxiety
- may get sweat rashes

Do you use/abuse drugs or drink alcohol excessively?
— no / yes →

drug or alcohol problem
- a sign, if you didn't already know it, that you may be a drug addict or alcoholic
- drugs or alcohol excess can cause sweating as can suddenly stopping or cutting down ('withdrawal')

Are you losing weight?
— no / yes →

overactive thyroid
- feel anxious/jumpy all the time
- lose weight despite eating well

or rare medical causes
e.g. TB, cancer

Only rare causes left, e.g.

medication side-effect

or serious illness

'Normal' Everything about the human body varies between individuals. Sweating is no exception: some people simply sweat more than others.

Treatment Not a lot you can do about normality, other than common-sense measures to keep the problem to a minimum – such as keeping cool, wearing light, loosely fitting clothes, and finding an effective antiperspirant.

Fever This is the body's response to an infection (usually a virus, such as flu). It pushes the temperature up to try to fight the germ off, and this causes sweating.

Treatment Regular paracetamol and plenty of cool fluids. The cause of the fever itself may need treating if it isn't a virus (see the 'High temperature' section, p. 65).

Anxiety It's obviously normal to feel anxious sometimes, in certain situations. In some people, this feeling is exaggerated, or stays most of the time. Sweating often accompanies anxiety of this sort.

Treatment This will depend on the cause of the anxiety (see 'Feeling tense' section). In general, burning off nervous energy through increased physical exercise, and trying relaxation therapy (such as relaxation tapes), often help.

Faint or near faint Faints are explained, and their treatment outlined, in the 'Loss of consciousness' section (p. 81). If you're about to faint, you may find you suddenly start to sweat – this stops when the faint is over.

Hypoglycaemia This is also explained in the 'Loss of consciousness' section (p. 81). As in fainting, sweating accompanies the attack.

Hyperhidrosis An overproduction of sweat on the palms and soles and in the armpits. It is simply an extreme of 'normal' but can be a real nuisance.

Treatment Strong antiperspirant roll-ons containing aluminium hexahydrate are available from the chemist. These especially help the armpits, but do less for the palms and soles. They can also cause dryness or itching of the skin, but this can, in turn, be treated with hydrocortisone 1% cream,

also available over the counter. If this fails and you're desperate, see your GP. There are some tablet treatments which can help, or he can refer you to a dermatologist for hospital-based treatment. Surgery is used as a last resort – this either involves removing the sweat-producing skin of the armpit or cutting the nerves which control the sweat glands in the palms.

Drug or alcohol abuse (or withdrawal) Drinking too much alcohol, or using illicit drugs such as amphetamines, can cause excess sweating. Stopping drugs (e.g. heroin) or alcohol suddenly leads to symptoms of withdrawal, when the body craves what it's missing. Sweating is a common sign of drug or alcohol withdrawal.

Treatment If you're having problems controlling the problem yourself, see your GP or local drug or alcohol advisory service for help.

Overactive thyroid The thyroid gland sits in the middle of the front of the neck, on and around the Adam's apple. It produces thyroid hormone, which controls the body's activity – too little and you slow up, too much and you feel overactive. The latter is called hyperthyroidism, and this can result in excessive sweating.

Treatment A GP job, as it requires a blood test to confirm the diagnosis – then, usually, referral to a specialist for treatment.

Medication side-effect A few prescribed treatments, such as antidepressants, can cause sweating as a side-effect – although sweating may also be caused by the problem the drug is trying to treat, like depression and anxiety.

Treatment If your GP thinks your problem is a side-effect of a treatment you are taking, he may be able to stop the drug or prescribe an alternative.

Rare medical causes Very rarely, persistent bouts of sweating, especially at night, are caused by serious illness such as TB, certain types of arthritis, or cancers of the immune system.

Treatment Your GP will arrange any necessary tests.

Feeling down

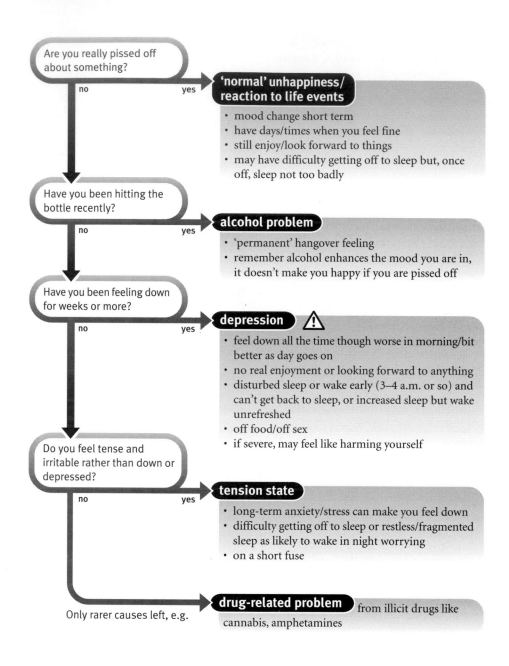

Are you really pissed off about something?

no   yes

'normal' unhappiness/ reaction to life events
- mood change short term
- have days/times when you feel fine
- still enjoy/look forward to things
- may have difficulty getting off to sleep but, once off, sleep not too badly

Have you been hitting the bottle recently?

no   yes

alcohol problem
- 'permanent' hangover feeling
- remember alcohol enhances the mood you are in, it doesn't make you happy if you are pissed off

Have you been feeling down for weeks or more?

no   yes

depression ⚠
- feel down all the time though worse in morning/bit better as day goes on
- no real enjoyment or looking forward to anything
- disturbed sleep or wake early (3–4 a.m. or so) and can't get back to sleep, or increased sleep but wake unrefreshed
- off food/off sex
- if severe, may feel like harming yourself

Do you feel tense and irritable rather than down or depressed?

no   yes

tension state
- long-term anxiety/stress can make you feel down
- difficulty getting off to sleep or restless/fragmented sleep as likely to wake in night worrying
- on a short fuse

Only rarer causes left, e.g.

drug-related problem from illicit drugs like cannabis, amphetamines

Remember: ⚠ means see your GP sharpish; ⚠ means an urgent hospital job

'Normal' unhappiness/reaction to life events

Short-term changes in mood are quite normal – some days, for no obvious reason, you're hacked off and others you've a spring in your step. Life crises will obviously get you down, but the misery they cause usually sorts itself out given time.

Treatment Time and the support of friends and family are the most helpful 'treatments'. Don't be tempted to turn to drink or drugs – they'll make matters worse. If you're having trouble coping, think about seeing your GP, who might arrange counselling – basically an opportunity to talk through your problems and emotions with someone trained to listen.

Alcohol problem

Overdoing the booze can cause depression in two ways – it has a direct chemical effect on the brain and, indirectly, it can create misery through a variety of social catastrophes, such as relationship problems or the loss of your driving licence.

Treatment Cut it down, or, better still, out. If you find this difficult, contact your local alcohol unit (try the Yellow Pages or ask at your doctor's surgery), or speak to your GP about the problem.

Depression

This is a feeling of low mood which lasts for weeks and which you just can't shake off. Other symptoms are usually present (see the chart). Sometimes, it's caused by a nasty life event, though it can start for no obvious reason. It's very common – estimates vary, but around one in twenty blokes will be suffering depression at any one time. Exactly what causes it isn't known, but many doctors now reckon it's linked to a lack of a certain chemical in the brain. When severe, it can make people extremely ill, or even suicidal.

Treatment Talk through your problems with your nearest and dearest and try the tips described for 'Tension state' (below). But if things aren't improving, see your GP. Counselling might help, or he may suggest antidepressants – this treatment really helps, is not addictive, and often has no significant side-effects. And it's a darn sight better than feeling crappy all the time. If you feel suicidal, seek medical help asap – or let those worried about you arrange for you to see the doc if you really can't see the point.

Tension state

A constant uptight feeling, usually linked to stress.

Treatment See if you can deal with whatever's winding you up and also try to get on top of the feeling of tension itself. For further details, see the 'Lifestyle/stress' part of the 'Feeling tense' section (p. 59).

Drug-related problem

Illicit drug use can cause a low mood. As with alcohol, the effect may be direct (long-term cannabis use can result in apathy, while stopping regular amphetamine use can cause symptoms of depression) or indirect, through a severely disrupted lifestyle.

Treatment Use the same approach as for alcohol – see above.

Feeling tense

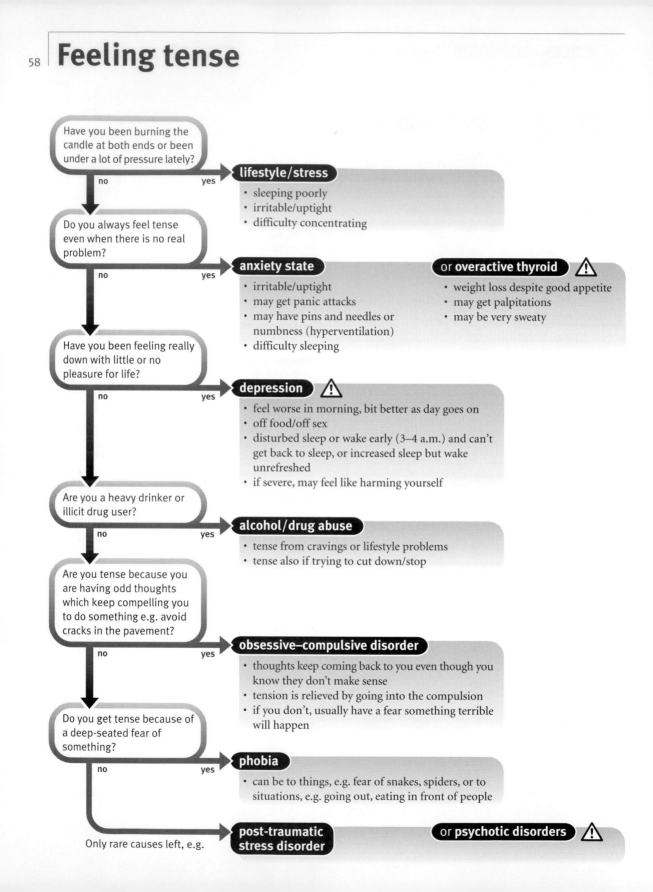

Have you been burning the candle at both ends or been under a lot of pressure lately?

no   yes

lifestyle/stress

- sleeping poorly
- irritable/uptight
- difficulty concentrating

Do you always feel tense even when there is no real problem?

no   yes

anxiety state

- irritable/uptight
- may get panic attacks
- may have pins and needles or numbness (hyperventilation)
- difficulty sleeping

or overactive thyroid

- weight loss despite good appetite
- may get palpitations
- may be very sweaty

Have you been feeling really down with little or no pleasure for life?

no   yes

depression

- feel worse in morning, bit better as day goes on
- off food/off sex
- disturbed sleep or wake early (3–4 a.m.) and can't get back to sleep, or increased sleep but wake unrefreshed
- if severe, may feel like harming yourself

Are you a heavy drinker or illicit drug user?

no   yes

alcohol/drug abuse

- tense from cravings or lifestyle problems
- tense also if trying to cut down/stop

Are you tense because you are having odd thoughts which keep compelling you to do something e.g. avoid cracks in the pavement?

no   yes

obsessive–compulsive disorder

- thoughts keep coming back to you even though you know they don't make sense
- tension is relieved by going into the compulsion
- if you don't, usually have a fear something terrible will happen

Do you get tense because of a deep-seated fear of something?

no   yes

phobia

- can be to things, e.g. fear of snakes, spiders, or to situations, e.g. going out, eating in front of people

Only rare causes left, e.g.

post-traumatic stress disorder

or psychotic disorders

Feeling tense

Lifestyle/stress Being under pressure – through, for example, relationship, work, or money worries – can make you feel uptight all the time.

Treatment If possible, try to get to the root of the problem by sorting out the stressful areas of your life. Increasing your physical exercise to burn off nervous energy, and cutting down your caffeine intake (e.g. tea, coffee, and cola) may help. Relaxation techniques are worthwhile: basically, this means whatever switches you off. If you're stuck, try a relaxation cassette tape or a self-help book – there are many available. You could also talk to your GP, as he might be able to advise you about other relaxation exercises, or send you to see someone to help manage your tension. But don't expect a prescription for a tranquillizer – these are hardly ever used these days.

Anxiety state A certain level of anxiety in certain circumstances is, of course, normal. But if feelings of anxiety are overwhelming, or continue when they should have settled, or appear for no reason, then they can become a problem. Also, an anxiety state can cause, or show itself through, 'panic attacks' (see the 'Hyperventilation' part of the 'Shortness of breath' section, p. 123).

Treatment The advice given in 'Lifestyle/stress' (above) may help (see also the treatment of panic attacks in the 'Shortness of breath' section, p. 123). If you're not able to get on top of the situation yourself, see your GP. He may be able to help by giving you some advice or by getting you to see someone who will teach you techniques to recognize and control your anxiety (such as a psychologist or a community psychiatric nurse). Tranquillizers are usually avoided if possible, although they may be used for a short while to ease a crisis.

Depression Depression and feeling tense often go hand in hand. For details about depression and its treatment, see the 'Feeling down' section (p. 57).

Alcohol/drug abuse Illicit substances may relax you while you're taking them, but usually end up making you tense – because your body may start to crave them, and because your lifestyle may become chaotic and difficult.

Treatment Cut them down or out. And if you're having problems, contact your GP or the local drug and alcohol unit.

Obsessive–compulsive disorder This is a psychological problem which has three parts. First, an obsession – a thought which keeps coming back to you even though you know it doesn't make sense (e.g. that your hands are covered in germs). Second, a compulsion, which is what the thought makes you do (keep washing your hands). And third, the feeling of tension that the whole thing creates. The cause is unknown.

Treatment If it's becoming a problem, see your GP. He'll either give you some advice or he may send you to see someone who specializes in this type of problem (such as a psychologist). Sometimes, medication is necessary and helpful.

Phobia This is an irrational fear which causes lots of worry. Well known examples include fear of open spaces (agoraphobia) and fear of spiders (arachnophobia). The cause is often unclear, though it may be linked to some upsetting event in your past.

Treatment If the phobia is a real problem, rather than a minor inconvenience, speak to your GP – he may be able to sort you out with some practical advice. Or you may need specialist help from someone skilled at helping people overcome phobias (usually a psychologist).

Post-traumatic stress disorder See the 'Problems sleeping' section (p. 111).

Overactive thyroid See the 'Excess sweating' section (p. 55). A feeling of tension is one of the many symptoms an overactive thyroid can produce.

Psychotic disorders These are illnesses like schizophrenia or mania. They cause a variety of symptoms, including, sometimes, a tension state. For further details, see the 'Odd behaviour' section (p. 95).

Hair loss

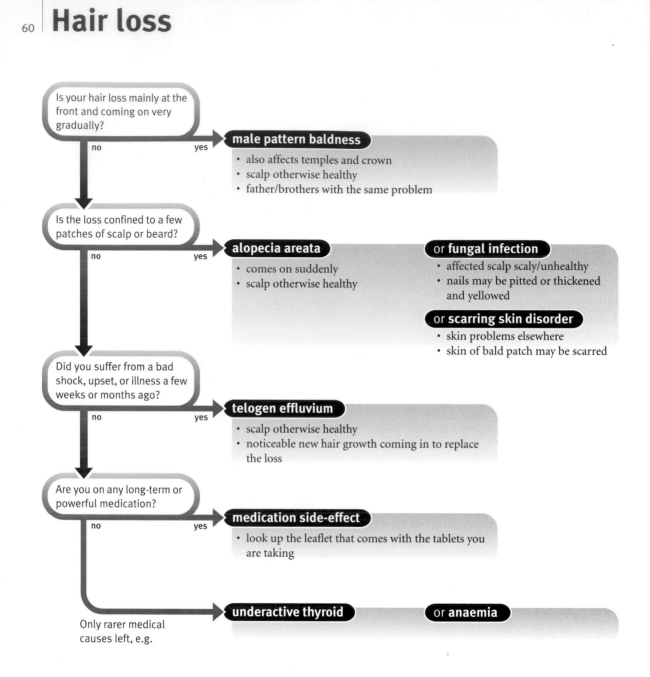

Is your hair loss mainly at the front and coming on very gradually?

no   yes

male pattern baldness
- also affects temples and crown
- scalp otherwise healthy
- father/brothers with the same problem

Is the loss confined to a few patches of scalp or beard?

no   yes

alopecia areata
- comes on suddenly
- scalp otherwise healthy

or fungal infection
- affected scalp scaly/unhealthy
- nails may be pitted or thickened and yellowed

or scarring skin disorder
- skin problems elsewhere
- skin of bald patch may be scarred

Did you suffer from a bad shock, upset, or illness a few weeks or months ago?

no   yes

telogen effluvium
- scalp otherwise healthy
- noticeable new hair growth coming in to replace the loss

Are you on any long-term or powerful medication?

no   yes

medication side-effect
- look up the leaflet that comes with the tablets you are taking

underactive thyroid   **or anaemia**

Only rarer medical causes left, e.g.

Male pattern baldness One of the disadvantages of being male is knowing that, sooner or later, you're likely to go bald: 5% of men are affected by the age of 20, rising to 80% by 70. The typical pattern affects the front, temple, and crown areas of the scalp. Blame your father: most men inherit their pattern of hair loss.

Treatment Beware – there are a huge number of so-called cures for baldness. Hardly any are worthwhile. Minoxidil, a cream available from the chemist, does help some men: it can cut down the amount of hair loss, but only causes good new growth in a minority. It is quite expensive, may take months to work, and if the treatment is stopped, any new hair which has grown may fall out. The only other effective treatments involve surgical techniques such as transplanting – a private and expensive business.

Alopecia areata Bald patches with a normal-looking scalp – it can also affect the beard area. The cause is unknown and it sometimes runs in families. Occasionally, it results in complete baldness – even, in extreme cases, loss of all body hair and problems with the nails too.

Treatment The good news is that the problem usually sorts itself out in time, usually over a year or so. The bad news is that, if it doesn't, treatment doesn't usually help much. You may be referred to a dermatologist, but more in hope than expectation: although treatments such as creams and injections into the scalp are often tried, their effects are usually very disappointing. Certain patterns of alopecia tend to last longest or get worse. These include people with several patches, loss of eyebrows and eyelashes, previous attacks, and loss of hair at the back of the head.

Telogen effluvium A human form of moulting. It is usually caused by some 'event' occurring about three months previously, such as a severe illness or psychological upset. As there is a delay of some months before the event leads to hair loss, a connection between the two often isn't made.

Treatment Don't waste your money or time on anything: your hair will be back to normal after about three months of moulting.

Medication side-effect Some treatments can cause hair loss. Most people know that powerful drugs given for cancer (chemotherapy) often result in baldness: you're highly unlikely to face this particular problem. Other drugs, such as blood thinning or anti-thyroid medications, can have the same effect.

Treatment If you think that a treatment you're taking is causing hair loss, discuss the situation with whoever is prescribing it – your GP or specialist.

Fungal infection Fungi – microscopic moulds – can get into the scalp and affect the hair. Commonly known as 'ringworm', the infection causes scaling with patches of baldness. It is much more common in children than adults.

Treatment See your GP for a course of anti-fungal pills.

Medical causes A variety of medical problems – such as anaemia and an underactive thyroid – can cause hair loss. The chances that these will come to light through baldness, though, is remote.

Treatment If your doc suspects a medical problem, he'll arrange the necessary blood tests and will treat you according to the results.

Scarring skin disorders Any skin diseases which cause scarring can lead to patches of hair loss – because hair won't grow where there are scars. These diseases are all very rare.

Treatment You're sure to be referred to a skin specialist for treatment.

Headache

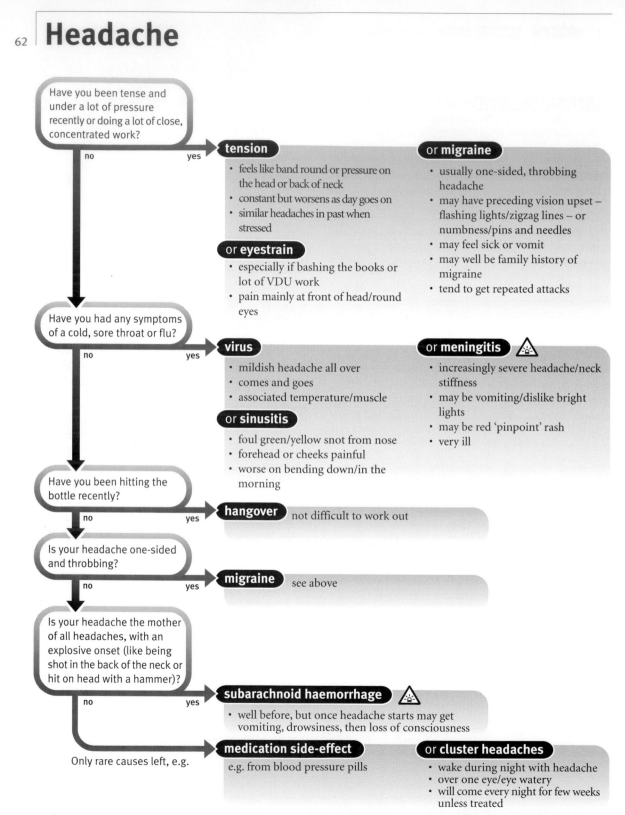

Have you been tense and under a lot of pressure recently or doing a lot of close, concentrated work?

no — yes →

tension
- feels like band round or pressure on the head or back of neck
- constant but worsens as day goes on
- similar headaches in past when stressed

or eyestrain
- especially if bashing the books or lot of VDU work
- pain mainly at front of head/round eyes

or migraine
- usually one-sided, throbbing headache
- may have preceding vision upset – flashing lights/zigzag lines – or numbness/pins and needles
- may feel sick or vomit
- may well be family history of migraine
- tend to get repeated attacks

Have you had any symptoms of a cold, sore throat or flu?

no — yes →

virus
- mildish headache all over
- comes and goes
- associated temperature/muscle

or sinusitis
- foul green/yellow snot from nose
- forehead or cheeks painful
- worse on bending down/in the morning

or meningitis ⚠
- increasingly severe headache/neck stiffness
- may be vomiting/dislike bright lights
- may be red 'pinpoint' rash
- very ill

Have you been hitting the bottle recently?

no — yes →

hangover not difficult to work out

Is your headache one-sided and throbbing?

no — yes →

migraine see above

Is your headache the mother of all headaches, with an explosive onset (like being shot in the back of the neck or hit on head with a hammer)?

no — yes →

subarachnoid haemorrhage ⚠
- well before, but once headache starts may get vomiting, drowsiness, then loss of consciousness

Only rare causes left, e.g.

medication side-effect
e.g. from blood pressure pills

or cluster headaches
- wake during night with headache
- over one eye/eye watery
- will come every night for few weeks unless treated

⚠ **If you get a sudden severe headache/pain in the back of your neck, or increasing headache and neck stiffness, seek medical help immediately to check for subarachnoid haemorrhage or meningitis.**

Headache

Virus A germ, causing a cold or flu. Headache is just part of the all-round grotty feeling that these germs cause.

Treatment Regular paracetamol or aspirin and plenty of fluids.

Tension headache Stress makes the muscles tense, especially on the forehead and in the neck. The tense muscles become tender, causing headache.

Treatment Massage, relaxation, and physical exercise will all help – see also the 'Feeling tense' section (p. 59). Avoid painkillers if possible as they can actually make it worse.

Hangover Figuring out why you've got a stonking headache – along with various other symptoms – the morning after the night before isn't exactly rocket science.

Treatment Dose yourself up with fluids (preferably fruit juice) and painkillers, and maybe some antacid if your stomach feels 'acidic'. Preventive measures in the future include avoiding binges and drinking plenty of water before crashing out.

Migraine Migraine is caused by the blood vessels to the brain opening wide – blood pumps through, causing a pounding headache. The cause is unknown, but it often runs in families, and attacks can be linked to diet, stress, or tiredness.

Treatment An attack of migraine needs rest and quiet, and strongish painkillers such as paracetamol and codeine combinations (available from the chemist without prescription). Soluble ones are often the most effective and quickest to work. If you get repeated attacks, try to figure out – and avoid – whatever brings them on. It's usually pretty obvious if it's something in your diet (such as cheese, chocolate, or red wine). Bear in mind that missing meals can also provoke attacks, so try to eat regularly. It's worth seeing your GP if the painkillers described above don't help or if you're getting very frequent attacks (say more than one a fortnight) – in both cases, he'll be able to prescribe treatment to help.

Sinusitis This is an infection of the sinuses, which are air spaces in your forehead and cheeks. The infection causes a build-up of pressure, resulting in pain over the affected sinus. If you tend to suffer a blocked nose most of the time, you might keep getting attacks of sinusitis.

Treatment Painkillers and steam inhalations, and see your GP if there's no improvement within a few days, as you may need antibiotics. You might also need some treatment to clear your nose if you keep getting attacks – being stuffed up all the time tends to block the sinuses, leading to repeated infections. This can be treated with either nose sprays or surgery.

Eyestrain If you can't see clearly, you'll tend to keep screwing your eyes up. This makes the muscles around the eyes sore, causing headache.

Treatment See an optician.

Cluster headache This is an unusual type of migraine which mainly affects blokes between the ages of 35 and 45.

Treatment See your GP for advice about what to take during an attack and possible preventative treatment.

Medication side-effect Some prescribed treatments, such as blood pressure pills, can cause headaches. Ironically, so can painkillers (even those bought over the counter) if used regularly.

Treatment Speak to your GP if you think a prescribed treatment is giving you headaches. And go easy on the painkillers.

Subarachnoid haemorrhage A burst blood vessel in the brain. Very serious and very rare.

Treatment Go straight to hospital.

Meningitis An infection of the lining of the brain. Also serious, but rarer than you'd think, considering the media coverage it gets.

Treatment This needs immediate attention. Call your doctor or go to hospital – whichever is likely to be quickest.

Other rare medical problems Some small print problems, including brain tumours and extremely high blood pressure, can cause headaches.

Treatment Problems like these are thankfully very rare, though the average patient is often worried about them by the time he decides to see his GP. So if you do visit the doc, anticipate lots of reassurance rather than a brain scan.

High temperature

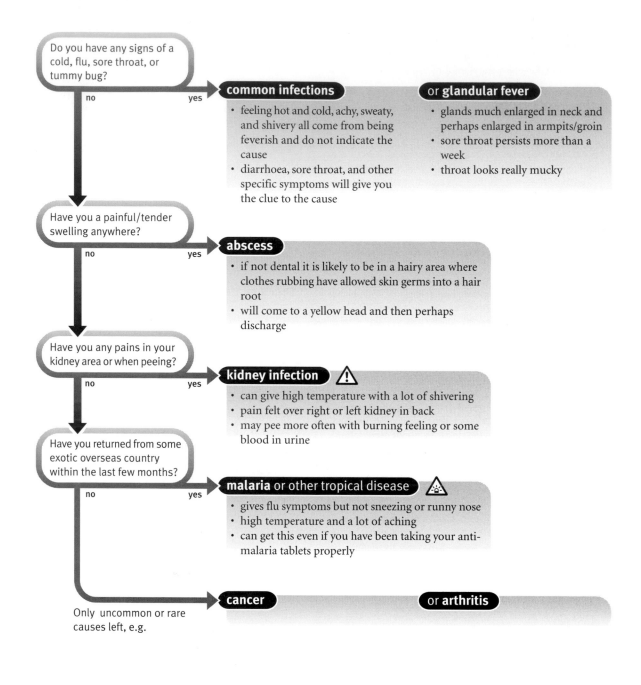

Do you have any signs of a cold, flu, sore throat, or tummy bug?

no / yes →

common infections

- feeling hot and cold, achy, sweaty, and shivery all come from being feverish and do not indicate the cause
- diarrhoea, sore throat, and other specific symptoms will give you the clue to the cause

or glandular fever

- glands much enlarged in neck and perhaps enlarged in armpits/groin
- sore throat persists more than a week
- throat looks really mucky

Have you a painful/tender swelling anywhere?

no / yes →

abscess

- if not dental it is likely to be in a hairy area where clothes rubbing have allowed skin germs into a hair root
- will come to a yellow head and then perhaps discharge

Have you any pains in your kidney area or when peeing?

no / yes →

kidney infection ⚠

- can give high temperature with a lot of shivering
- pain felt over right or left kidney in back
- may pee more often with burning feeling or some blood in urine

Have you returned from some exotic overseas country within the last few months?

no / yes →

malaria or other tropical disease ⚠

- gives flu symptoms but not sneezing or runny nose
- high temperature and a lot of aching
- can get this even if you have been taking your anti-malaria tablets properly

Only uncommon or rare causes left, e.g.

cancer   or arthritis

Remember: ⚠ means see your GP sharpish; ⚠ means an urgent hospital job

Common infections These include colds, tonsillitis, chest infections, flu, and tummy bugs, which can all cause a high temperature for a few days. Pushing your temperature up is actually one of the ways your body tries to fight off these germs – the fever fries the bug and also makes your immune defences work faster.

Treatment The temperature itself needs no treatment at all, though you'll feel more comfortable if you keep yourself as cool as possible and take regular paracetamol and plenty of fluids. Otherwise, it's a question of sorting out the infection which is causing the high temperature. Most (including colds, the flu, and most tummy bugs) are caused by viruses, which usually settle on their own in a few days – there's no magic cure for these infections. Some, such as tonsillitis and chest infections, may be helped by antibiotics (see the 'Sore throat', p. 127 and 'Cough' sections, p. 43).

Glandular fever This is explained, and its treatment outlined, in the 'Sore throat' section (p. 127).

Abscess Abscesses are infections which develop into lumps of pus, like very large and painful boils. They can appear anywhere on the body, especially in hairy areas and around the back passage. They can also develop inside the body – this is much more unusual, but can happen, for example, after a severe chest or kidney infection. Your temperature will tend to go up and down until the abscess clears up.

Treatment An early abscess may be cured by antibiotics. Otherwise, it'll need lancing – see your GP or go to casualty. Internal abscesses are obviously more complicated and need hospital treatment, which your GP will arrange.

Kidney infection A germ getting into your kidney will push your temperature up and cause other symptoms too. This is pretty unusual and can be a sign of some other problem with your waterworks, such as kidney stones.

Treatment You need to see your GP asap for treatment with antibiotics. Drinking plenty of fluids will help too. If you're really rough with it, and vomiting, you may need to go to hospital. You may also need further tests once you're better to work out why you developed a kidney infection in the first place.

Malaria (and other tropical diseases) People very occasionally bring back exotic illnesses as unpleasant souvenirs of their travels abroad. A few of these – and some types of malaria in particular – develop slowly and may cause a high temperature which keeps coming back, before any other symptoms develop.

Treatment If you've been somewhere exotic and you've developed a persistent fever which has no obvious cause (like a cold or sore throat), see your GP asap, especially if you feel really rough too. Do this even if you've taken anti-malaria pills or it's been some months since you travelled: malaria can take quite a while to develop, and the pills taken to prevent it aren't 100% effective. Besides, you may have some exotic infection other than malaria. If your GP thinks you may have brought home an unusual germ of this sort, he'll either arrange some urgent blood tests or send you to hospital.

Cancer Any cancer can cause a recurring high temperature. An example is lymphoma (see the 'Swollen glands' section, p. 139). Most other cancers produce other symptoms which give the game away.

Treatment It's most unlikely that your temperature is caused by anything nasty – but if you're worried, see your GP.

Rare infections Some serious and unusual infections, such as meningitis and septicaemia (blood poisoning), can cause a sudden high temperature as your body tries to fight them off. There are likely to be other symptoms too, and you'll be feeling seriously ill. Some other rare but important infections don't come on so dramatically. Examples include TB and infection with the HIV virus (the cause of AIDS). These type of germs can cause a prolonged or recurrent fever and usually make you feel gradually more unwell.

Treatment Meningitis and blood poisoning require immediate treatment in hospital. If you're worried you might have TB or HIV infection, you need to see your GP soon to discuss the situation – he will arrange any necessary tests.

Arthritis Rheumatoid arthritis and some other rare types of arthritis – but not the common 'wear and tear' sort (osteoarthritis) – can give you a recurrent high temperature, amongst other symptoms.

Treatment See your GP. He will refer you to a joint specialist (a rheumatologist). For further information, see the 'Rheumatoid arthritis' part of the 'Multiple joint pains' section (p. 89).

Other uncommon medical conditions Problems which can very occasionally cause a prolonged temperature include inflammatory bowel disease (see the 'Diarrhoea' section, p. 47) and the side-effects of medication.

Treatment Talk to your GP if you think you might have one of these rare causes.

Hoarse voice

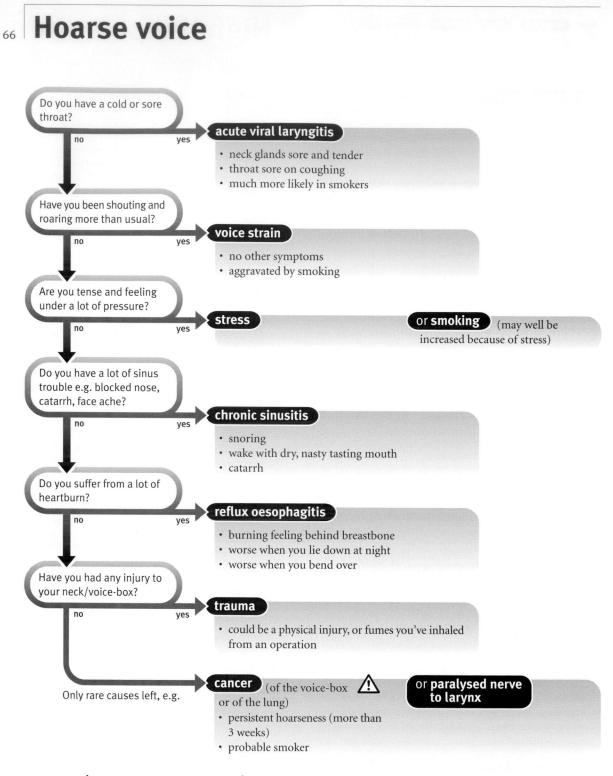

Do you have a cold or sore throat?

no / **yes**

acute viral laryngitis
- neck glands sore and tender
- throat sore on coughing
- much more likely in smokers

Have you been shouting and roaring more than usual?

no / **yes**

voice strain
- no other symptoms
- aggravated by smoking

Are you tense and feeling under a lot of pressure?

no / **yes**

stress   **or smoking** (may well be increased because of stress)

Do you have a lot of sinus trouble e.g. blocked nose, catarrh, face ache?

no / **yes**

chronic sinusitis
- snoring
- wake with dry, nasty tasting mouth
- catarrh

Do you suffer from a lot of heartburn?

no / **yes**

reflux oesophagitis
- burning feeling behind breastbone
- worse when you lie down at night
- worse when you bend over

Have you had any injury to your neck/voice-box?

no / **yes**

trauma
- could be a physical injury, or fumes you've inhaled from an operation

Only rare causes left, e.g.

cancer (of the voice-box ⚠ or of the lung)   **or paralysed nerve to larynx**
- persistent hoarseness (more than 3 weeks)
- probable smoker

Remember: ⚠ means see your GP sharpish; ⚠ means an urgent hospital job

Acute viral laryngitis The common germs which cause colds and sore throats can inflame the voice-box (or larynx), causing hoarseness.

Treatment Try some simple self-help measures like hot drinks, steam inhalations, and paracetamol while you're waiting the few days for the problem to settle. Also, avoid cigarette smoke and go easy on your voice – so no shouting or lengthy phone conversations. Antibiotics don't usually help this problem, but, if you also get a bad cough with a lot of green or yellow spit, you may be developing a chest infection (see 'Cough' section, p. 43) which might be helped by a short course.

Voice strain There are two types. The 'acute' sort simply means you've strained your voice-box by screaming or shouting. You don't need a doctor to tell you that hurling abuse from the terraces, or shouting to make yourself heard at a party, can leave you hoarse for a day or two. The 'chronic' sort is caused by continuous voice strain – such as untrained singing – and makes the voice hoarse, to some extent, most of the time. Sometimes, this can result in small lumps ('singers' nodules') on the vocal cords.

Treatment Chronic voice strain will only be cured if you either stop whatever is upsetting your voice-box, or start doing it properly. So if you're a singer with this problem, try getting some voice training. If the hoarseness has been there for ages, and continues despite your best efforts, you might have singer's nodules. Ear, Nose, and Throat ('ENT') surgeons can deal with these quite easily, so discuss the situation with your GP.

Smoking Cigarette smoke irritates the vocal cords, making them swell slightly. This can make the voice constantly hoarse.

Treatment Stopping smoking should sort the problem out, unless you're also abusing your vocal cords in some other way (see 'Voice strain', above).

Stress Small muscles in the voice-box help produce the sounds of your voice. If you're uptight, these muscles get tense and so don't produce the sounds properly. This usually happens in certain stressful situations, like making a speech or giving a presentation; sometimes, if you're very tense all the time, the voice tends to stay hoarse.

Treatment Try the relaxation advice given in the 'Anxiety'

part of the 'Palpitations' section (p. 103). Voice training may help if your voice only lets you down in certain stressful situations.

Chronic sinusitis The sinuses are air spaces in the skull. If you have some problem with your nose – such as a blockage caused by polyps, allergy, or an old injury – the drainage system of the sinuses may not work properly. This causes the sinuses to fill with fluid, which gets infected and tends to drip down the back of the throat, causing catarrh and an inflamed voice-box.

Treatment Self-help measures include steam inhalations and stopping smoking. If your nose is blocked or runs a lot of the time, you could try an anti-allergy nose spray from the chemist such as beclomethasone. If you're getting nowhere and the symptom is a real nuisance, see your GP – he may try some other treatments or he may refer you to an ENT surgeon for possible surgery to unblock your nose.

Trauma Any damage to the voice-box will cause hoarseness. Possibilities include a punch, accidentally breathing in hot steam or chemical fumes, and any operation under anaesthetic (because of the large tube put down your throat during surgery).

Treatment The hoarseness will right itself after a few days. Seek medical attention urgently if a blow to the throat, or inhaling something nasty, is making it hard to breathe.

Damaged nerve to larynx If this nerve is damaged, then one or both of your vocal cords will be paralysed. This has a number of very rare causes.

Treatment Your GP is certain to send you to an, ENT specialist to get the problem sorted out.

Reflux oesophagitis This is explained in the 'Indigestion' section. It can result in hoarseness if the acid comes right up the gullet into the voice-box, where it causes an irritation.

Treatment See the 'Indigestion' section (p. 71).

Cancer Highly unlikely in the under 50s, and incredibly unlikely in non-smokers.

Treatment See your GP, who will send you for an urgent appointment at the hospital if he's concerned.

Impotence

NB Impotence is an inability to get – or keep – a proper erection. For information about the problem of going off sex, see the 'Loss of sex drive' section.

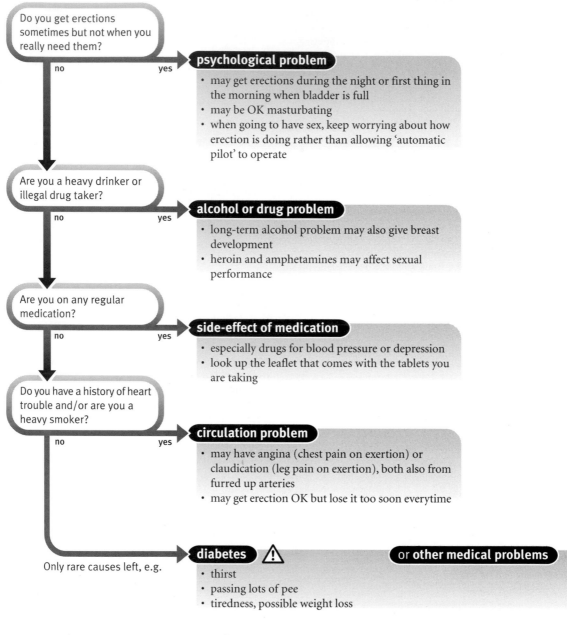

Do you get erections sometimes but not when you really need them?

no / yes

psychological problem
- may get erections during the night or first thing in the morning when bladder is full
- may be OK masturbating
- when going to have sex, keep worrying about how erection is doing rather than allowing 'automatic pilot' to operate

Are you a heavy drinker or illegal drug taker?

no / yes

alcohol or drug problem
- long-term alcohol problem may also give breast development
- heroin and amphetamines may affect sexual performance

Are you on any regular medication?

no / yes

side-effect of medication
- especially drugs for blood pressure or depression
- look up the leaflet that comes with the tablets you are taking

Do you have a history of heart trouble and/or are you a heavy smoker?

no / yes

circulation problem
- may have angina (chest pain on exertion) or claudication (leg pain on exertion), both also from furred up arteries
- may get erection OK but lose it too soon everytime

Only rare causes left, e.g.

diabetes ⚠
- thirst
- passing lots of pee
- tiredness, possible weight loss

or other medical problems

Remember: ⚠ means see your GP sharpish; ⚠ means an urgent hospital job

Psychological problems If you get erections at certain times (e.g. early morning) then your tackle must be in good working order – so the problem is above the neck rather than below the waist. Maybe you're just very tired or stressed. Maybe you just don't fancy your partner any more, or you're feeling guilty about a fling, or you're worried about getting her pregnant. Whatever the reason, a vicious circle soon builds up: the fear of another sexual flop breeds more stress, resulting in further failure. This is known as 'performance anxiety' and it tends to aggravate the situation, whatever the original problem.

Treatment It's normal for your tackle to underperform if you're simply knackered or uptight about something. If the problem persists, try to sort out the underlying cause, whether it's a relationship problem, stress, or whatever. This may be difficult, but at least get the issue out in the open by discussing it fully and frankly with your partner. This in itself may help to sort it out and will, at least, defuse the performance anxiety. If you're getting nowhere check out one of the many helpful books devoted to the subject, or see your GP – he may be able to help, or he may refer you and your partner for psychosexual counselling (which basically means talking it through with a sexpert). Alternatively, he may prescribe you a treatment to help you get an erection, such as Viagra. Although this doesn't get to the root of your psychological problem, it can break the vicious cycle described above, which may be a 'kick-start' to getting yourself sorted out.

Alcohol or drug problem In the short term, a boozing binge can lead to the dreaded brewer's droop. In the longer term, heavy drinking can cause sexual problems by blocking the male hormones. Some illicit drugs – for example, heroin and amphetamines – can also cause impotence.

Treatment Reduce, or, better still, stop the booze or drugs. Discuss with your GP if you're having problems doing this, or you succeed but it doesn't solve the problem.

Medication side-effect Some prescribed treatments can cause impotence. The most likely culprits include antidepressants and blood pressure pills.

Treatment Check out the leaflet in the packaging of your treatment. If sexual problems or impotence are listed, discuss the situation with your GP – he may be able to stop the treatment or suggest an alternative.

Circulation problem When you get an erection, your penis may feel like it's throbbing with blood. That's because it is. If the blood vessels supplying the penis get furred up, it can be difficult for enough blood to get through to cause – or keep – an erection. Smoking is the likely cause, as this clogs up the arteries; it also narrows them by putting them into spasm. Erection problems can also be caused by the veins of the penis draining the blood away too quickly.

Treatment The key is giving up smoking. Remember to discuss the problem too (see above). If there's no improvement after a few months, see your GP – he may want to check out your circulation, run a few tests, refer you to a specialist, or try a treatment like Viagra.

Diabetes If your body fails to produce enough of the chemical 'insulin', your blood sugar starts to rise: this is diabetes. It's quite common, affecting one in a hundred people, but no one knows exactly why it happens. The high sugar level in your blood can cause a number of problems, including impotence. If you already know you're diabetic, then this is quite likely to be the cause of your impotence.

Treatment See your doc asap – and take a specimen of wee with you, as he'll want to test this. If it does turn out that you have diabetes, you'll need a special diet, probably with either tablets or insulin injections. And if you already know you have diabetes, pluck up the courage to book an appointment to see your GP. Getting your blood sugar under control may solve the problem; if not, then he might prescribe you a treatment such as Viagra which is likely to help.

Other medical problems A load of small print stuff involving nerve supplies and hormones which you'll almost certainly not need to worry about.

Treatment Make an appointment with your GP so he can rule out any rarities.

Indigestion

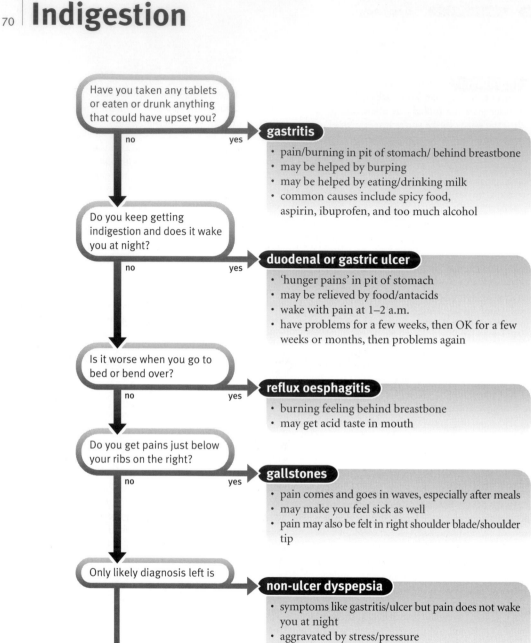

Have you taken any tablets or eaten or drunk anything that could have upset you?

no | yes

gastritis
- pain/burning in pit of stomach/ behind breastbone
- may be helped by burping
- may be helped by eating/drinking milk
- common causes include spicy food, aspirin, ibuprofen, and too much alcohol

Do you keep getting indigestion and does it wake you at night?

no | yes

duodenal or gastric ulcer
- 'hunger pains' in pit of stomach
- may be relieved by food/antacids
- wake with pain at 1–2 a.m.
- have problems for a few weeks, then OK for a few weeks or months, then problems again

Is it worse when you go to bed or bend over?

no | yes

reflux oesphagitis
- burning feeling behind breastbone
- may get acid taste in mouth

Do you get pains just below your ribs on the right?

no | yes

gallstones
- pain comes and goes in waves, especially after meals
- may make you feel sick as well
- pain may also be felt in right shoulder blade/shoulder tip

Only likely diagnosis left is

non-ulcer dyspepsia
- symptoms like gastritis/ulcer but pain does not wake you at night
- aggravated by stress/pressure
- may have irritable bowel with tummy gripes/ diarrhoea when stressed

Or rare cause, e.g.

cancer of the stomach ⚠
- vague indigestion symptoms
- may lose appetite/feel sick
- may lose weight

Indigestion

Gastritis The stomach produces acid to help digest the food. But sometimes the acid can inflame the stomach lining ('gastritis'), causing indigestion. There are a number of things which can stir up acid problems. The commonest is alcohol – this is why indigestion is a familiar part of a hangover. Some tablets, such as aspirin and anti-inflammatory drugs (like ibuprofen), can have the same effect.

Treatment If this is a one-off problem – such as after an alcohol binge – just drink plenty of water and take some antacids from the chemist. But if you keep getting problems, look at your diet and lifestyle. Avoid spicy foods, eat regularly, and cut down cigarettes and booze. Also, steer clear of acidic over-the-counter painkillers like aspirin and ibuprofen; paracetamol is OK. Antacids – used when needed – are usually very helpful.

Duodenal or gastric ulcer Occasionally, the acid burns a small crater in the lining of the tube which carries food away from the stomach (a duodenal ulcer) or, less commonly, in the stomach itself (a gastric ulcer). This type of problem sometimes runs in families and may be brought on, or aggravated by, the things discussed above.

Treatment This is explained in the 'Gastritis/ulcer' part of the 'Abdominal pain – recurrent' section (p. 15).

Non-ulcer dyspepsia This gives all the symptoms of acidity or ulcers but is caused by something else – probably the muscles of the stomach and gullet squeezing too hard or in an uncoordinated way. So it's a bit like 'irritable bowel syndrome' (see the 'Abdominal pain – recurrent' section, p. 15). In fact, many people with non-ulcer dyspepsia also get irritable bowel syndrome, and some doctors think they're actually the same thing. The cause is unknown, but it may be linked to stress.

Treatment It's sensible to look at the lifestyle areas discussed above. Antacids do seem to help some people, even though it's not really caused by excess acid. If your symptoms do seem to be stress related, try to sort out whatever is winding you up and do some relaxation therapy (see the 'Feeling tense' section, p. 59). It's worth seeing your GP if you're getting nowhere: he might try more powerful acid-suppressant pills or medication to relax the muscles in your stomach and gullet. There may be no 'magic bullet', though, so you may have to accept that you'll get some symptoms from time to time.

Reflux oesophagitis Acid sits in the stomach, waiting to digest food, and is prevented from entering the gullet by a valve. If this valve doesn't work perfectly, the acid can rise into the gullet, inflaming its lining ('reflux oesophagitis'). This is usually felt as a burning in the centre of the chest ('heartburn'), which can lead to indigestion.

Treatment You can make a variety of tweaks to your lifestyle which should help. These include: shedding some pounds if you're overweight; taking care not to overdo the spicy foods and alcohol; cutting down, or stopping, smoking; not eating too late in the evening; raising the head of your bed by a few inches; and avoiding acidic over-the-counter painkillers like aspirin and ibuprofen. Antacid mixtures from the chemist can help if you get a lot of heartburn; if they don't work, more powerful treatments are available from your GP.

Gallstones These are discussed, and their treatment explained, in the 'Abdominal pain – one-off' section (p. 13). They can cause an indigestion-type pain, especially after fatty meals.

Stomach cancer Relax. This is rare in the under 50s.

Treatment It's extremely unlikely that you've got this problem unless you're over 50. Speak to your GP if you're concerned. If he's in any doubt, he'll arrange for a specialist at the hospital to take a look into your stomach with a narrow, flexible telescope (called an 'endoscope').

Infertility

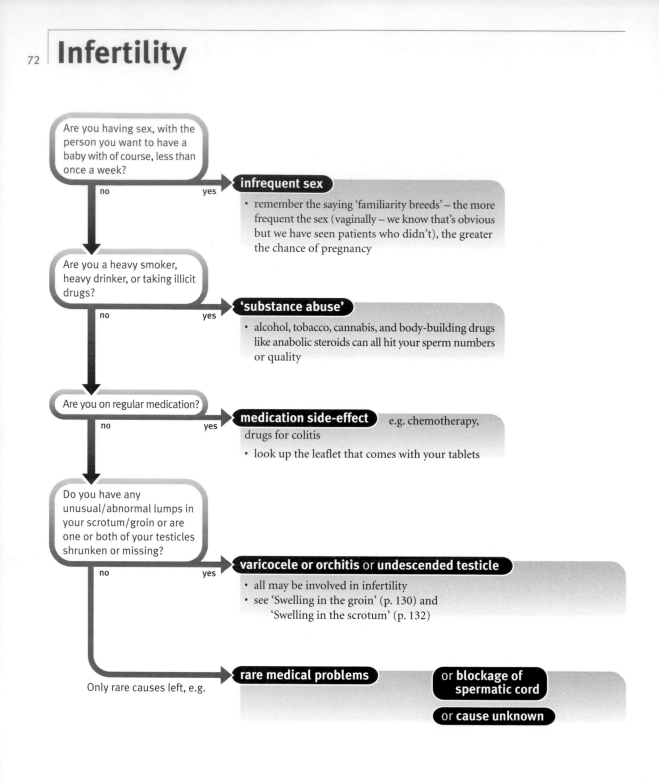

Are you having sex, with the person you want to have a baby with of course, less than once a week?

no / yes

infrequent sex

- remember the saying 'familiarity breeds' – the more frequent the sex (vaginally – we know that's obvious but we have seen patients who didn't), the greater the chance of pregnancy

Are you a heavy smoker, heavy drinker, or taking illicit drugs?

no / yes

'substance abuse'

- alcohol, tobacco, cannabis, and body-building drugs like anabolic steroids can all hit your sperm numbers or quality

Are you on regular medication?

no / yes

medication side-effect e.g. chemotherapy, drugs for colitis

- look up the leaflet that comes with your tablets

Do you have any unusual/abnormal lumps in your scrotum/groin or are one or both of your testicles shrunken or missing?

no / yes

varicocele or orchitis or **undescended testicle**

- all may be involved in infertility
- see 'Swelling in the groin' (p. 130) and 'Swelling in the scrotum' (p. 132)

rare medical problems

Only rare causes left, e.g.

or blockage of spermatic cord

or cause unknown

Remember: ⚠ means see your GP sharpish; ⚠ means an urgent hospital job

NB 1. For fertility problems caused by impotence or ejaculation trouble, see the 'Impotence' (p. 68) and 'Problems with ejaculation' (p. 114) sections.

2. Most couples will manage to achieve a pregnancy within a year of trying – and those who don't usually succeed in the second year. But about one in seven couples have difficulty. It's often caused by a combination of problems in both the man and the woman, rather than the cause lying with one or the other – so it's best to view it as a joint problem and, if you opt to see the doc, to go together. In about a third of cases, the bloke is found to be infertile or subfertile.

Cause unknown To get your partner pregnant you need plenty of active, healthy sperm. In 60% of cases, the cause of lousy sperm remains a mystery.

Treatment If you've been trying for ages without success, the usual form is that your GP will arrange for you to have a sperm test. This analyses your sperm under the microscope, checking their number and how healthy and active they are – duff sperm are scanty, or sluggish, or abnormal looking. Don't despair if you're told that the result isn't great. It'll need repeating in a few months because sperm counts vary from time to time, and can be affected by illnesses like the flu. Your second test may be a lot better. If it isn't, your GP is likely to refer you and your partner to a specialist.

Infrequent sex Obviously, if pressure of work, night shifts, or frequent travel mean that you're limited to the very occasional bonk, you're lowering your chances of getting your partner pregnant, regardless of your sperm count.

Treatment Just what you've always wanted the doc to order – more frequent sex. But try to avoid the ritual of 'timed' sex using fertility gizmos, as this tends to result in stress and a screwed-up love life.

Alcohol, tobacco, cannabis, & anabolic steroids

Not such good news. All these pleasures or enhancers can significantly affect your sperm – enough to tip the balance into infertility problems.

Treatment Cut down or give up whatever is likely to be spiking your sperm.

Medication side-effect A few prescribed treatments (such as chemotherapy and some treatments for colitis) can affect your sperm count.

Treatment Hopefully, you'll have been warned about this before you started the treatment so that you'll have had a chance to produce a sperm sample which can be frozen and stored for future use. If not, and you think your treatment might be affecting your fertility, discuss the situation with your doctor.

Varicocele This is explained, and the treatment discussed, in the 'Swelling in the scrotum' section (p. 133).

Orchitis See the 'Pain in the testicle' section (p. 101). Orchitis affecting only one testicle does not cause fertility problems; if it affects both sides, and makes the testicles shrink, it can affect the sperm count enough to cause infertility, though this is rare.

Blockage of spermatic cord Previous infection (especially sexually transmitted germs) can sometimes block the spermatic cord, which takes the sperm from the testicle to the penis.

Treatment If you have a blocked spermatic cord, your GP will refer you to a hospital consultant for surgery to bypass the block, or other specialized treatment.

Undescended testicle See the 'Undescended testicle' part of the 'Swelling in the groin' section (p. 131). If you had this problem as a child, your testicle may end up not producing sperm properly.

Treatment If maldescent of your testicle has made you infertile, your GP will refer you and your partner to a specialist for further help.

(**Rare medical problems**) Serious illnesses, such as kidney or liver disease and problems with the glands which produce your hormones, can cause infertility.

Treatment It's very unlikely that these problems will come to light through infertility – it's much more likely that you're already known to have the medical problem and that infertility is just one part of it. But if you are worried about your general state of health, and you're having trouble getting your partner pregnant, discuss the situation with your GP.

Itchy scalp

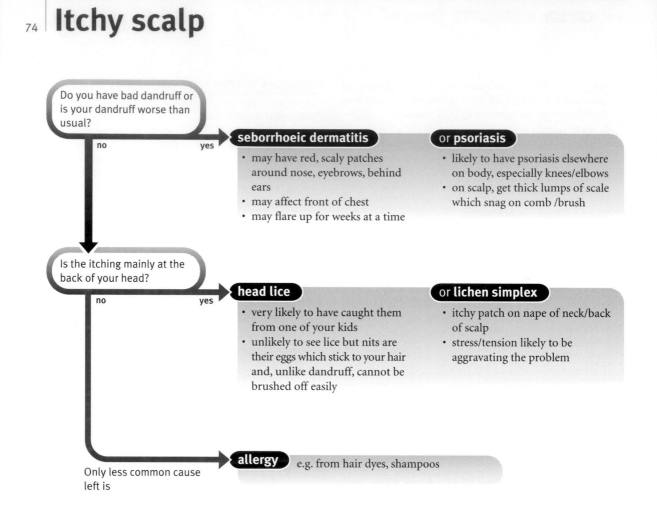

Do you have bad dandruff or is your dandruff worse than usual?

no | yes

seborrhoeic dermatitis
- may have red, scaly patches around nose, eyebrows, behind ears
- may affect front of chest
- may flare up for weeks at a time

or psoriasis
- likely to have psoriasis elsewhere on body, especially knees/elbows
- on scalp, get thick lumps of scale which snag on comb /brush

Is the itching mainly at the back of your head?

no | yes

head lice
- very likely to have caught them from one of your kids
- unlikely to see lice but nits are their eggs which stick to your hair and, unlike dandruff, cannot be brushed off easily

or lichen simplex
- itchy patch on nape of neck/back of scalp
- stress/tension likely to be aggravating the problem

Only less common cause left is

allergy e.g. from hair dyes, shampoos

Seborrhoeic dermatitis This is a type of eczema of the scalp caused by an infection with a fungus, which makes the scalp dry, flaky, itchy, and sometimes sore. Dandruff is caused by seborrhoeic dermatitis, which, if mild, leads to some flaking of the scalp but little, if any, itch.

Treatment If you've just got mild dandruff, regular hair washing with an anti-dandruff or anti-fungal shampoo should sort it out. Coal tar-based shampoos are good for the itching but won't get rid of the underlying problem. If you're having terrible problems with dandruff and irritation, see your GP – he can prescribe very effective anti-fungal and anti-itch shampoos and lotions. Seborrhoeic dermatitis can keep coming back, so you may need to repeat the treatment from time to time.

Psoriasis This can affect various parts of the body, including the scalp. It produces a patchy, scaly rash which sometimes gets itchy. On the scalp, the skin gets very thick and roughened, leading to bad dandruff. The cause is unknown, but it sometimes runs in families.

Treatment Strong coal tar shampoos (available from the chemist) can help. Otherwise, you'll need to discuss the situation with your GP, who can prescribe various shampoos or lotions to ease the problem. It can be difficult to sort out and you may need to try a lot of different treatments before you strike lucky – and, like seborrhoeic dermatitis, it can keep coming back. If you have really severe scalp psoriasis and nothing seems to help, your GP may refer you to a dermatologist (a skin specialist).

Head lice Lice are tiny insects which can live in your hair – the severe itch is caused by the bites they inflict on your scalp as they suck blood. The problem is much commoner in children but can occur in adults and is passed on by close contact or by sharing brushes or combs. Another type of louse prefers your pubes (often called 'crabs') – this one is usually passed on by having sex with an infected partner.

Treatment Get an anti-lice lotion and/or bug-busting comb from the chemist and follow the instructions very closely. And make sure you check your household contacts for lice too, otherwise you'll get infected again (look for nits, which are tiny lice eggs attached near the base of hairs, especially behind the ears – you can tell they're not dandruff because they're quite hard to separate from the hairs). If you've got crabs, apply a lotion from the chemist to your pubic hairs. Check other hairy areas too, as the little buggers can spread, even to eyebrows and eyelashes; and, of course, enquire delicately whether or not your partner has noticed any wildlife crawling around her undergrowth.

Lichen simplex This is an itchy patch usually found on the nape of the neck and the back of the scalp. It's probably caused by stress: being tense makes you scratch or rub the back of your head, which inflames the skin and which, in turn, causes itching and so more scratching – and so it continues.

Treatment Coal tar shampoos and hydrocortisone 1% cream from the chemist can help relieve the irritation – or you may need something stronger from your GP. But you won't cure the problem unless you stop scratching or rubbing the affected area. Try to sort out whatever's stressing you and check out some of the relaxation measures discussed in the 'Feeling tense' section.

Allergy Occasionally, your scalp can get inflamed because of an allergy to something you've put on it. The likeliest culprits are hair dyes (if you go in for that type of thing) and shampoos.

Treatment The problem will sort itself out in a couple of days. Make sure you avoid whatever's brought it on in future.

Itchy skin

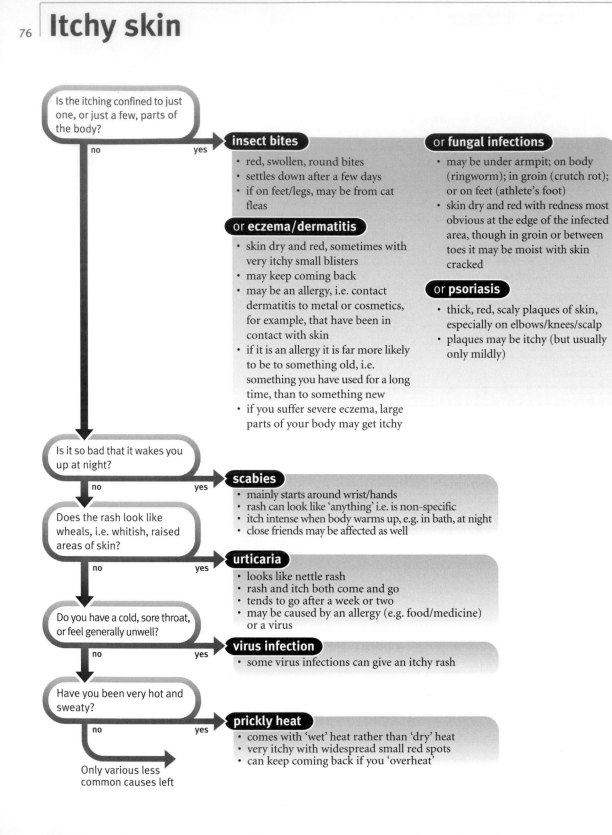

Is the itching confined to just one, or just a few, parts of the body?

no / **yes**

insect bites
- red, swollen, round bites
- settles down after a few days
- if on feet/legs, may be from cat fleas

or **eczema/dermatitis**
- skin dry and red, sometimes with very itchy small blisters
- may keep coming back
- may be an allergy, i.e. contact dermatitis to metal or cosmetics, for example, that have been in contact with skin
- if it is an allergy it is far more likely to be to something old, i.e. something you have used for a long time, than to something new
- if you suffer severe eczema, large parts of your body may get itchy

or **fungal infections**
- may be under armpit; on body (ringworm); in groin (crutch rot); or on feet (athlete's foot)
- skin dry and red with redness most obvious at the edge of the infected area, though in groin or between toes it may be moist with skin cracked

or **psoriasis**
- thick, red, scaly plaques of skin, especially on elbows/knees/scalp
- plaques may be itchy (but usually only mildly)

Is it so bad that it wakes you up at night?

no / **yes**

scabies
- mainly starts around wrist/hands
- rash can look like 'anything' i.e. is non-specific
- itch intense when body warms up, e.g. in bath, at night
- close friends may be affected as well

Does the rash look like wheals, i.e. whitish, raised areas of skin?

no / **yes**

urticaria
- looks like nettle rash
- rash and itch both come and go
- tends to go after a week or two
- may be caused by an allergy (e.g. food/medicine) or a virus

Do you have a cold, sore throat, or feel generally unwell?

no / **yes**

virus infection
- some virus infections can give an itchy rash

Have you been very hot and sweaty?

no / **yes**

prickly heat
- comes with 'wet' heat rather than 'dry' heat
- very itchy with widespread small red spots
- can keep coming back if you 'overheat'

Only various less common causes left

Insect bites Bites from insects produce a characteristic itchy rash.

Treatment Calamine lotion and antihistamine tablets (see below) will ease the problem. And if you have a cat or dog at home, get it checked for fleas.

Eczema/dermatitis This means inflamed skin – it becomes red, itchy, and dry or weepy. There are many different types, each with characteristic patterns. In most cases, the cause is unknown, but a few result from allergy (such as an allergy to the nickel in your jeans buckle or your metal watch strap – but almost never an allergy to something you've eaten). Some start in childhood (especially the type which is linked with hay fever and asthma) and others only appear when you're older.

Treatment This is pretty much the same whatever your type of eczema. First of all, look after your skin: wash regularly but avoid perfumed soaps or bubble baths, and, if your hands are affected, keep them out of detergents – if you must do the washing up, wear rubber gloves (make sure they've got a cotton lining because rubber can aggravate the problem). Moisturiser is important if your skin is dry. You can get various types from the chemist (such as aqueous cream); some people use this as a soap substitute too. It's also worth using a mild steroid cream – hydrocortisone 1% is available over the counter and is perfectly safe to use, even on the face. Bear in mind that these treatments only ease, rather than cure, the problem – unfortunately, eczema can keep coming back, and it's just a case of using the treatments whenever it flares up. Don't mess around with your diet, either, as this almost never helps. If the pattern of your eczema suggests an allergy then avoid whatever you think might be bringing it on. And if you've tried all the measures described without much effect, see your GP – he'll be able to prescribe you other treatments to get on top of the problem.

Scabies This is caused by a microscopic insect which burrows into the skin. The rash is actually an allergy to the insect's droppings, and can be incredibly itchy. It is passed on by close contact but may take a few weeks to develop.

Treatment You can get anti-scabies lotions from the chemist. It's vital that you read the instructions carefully and apply it exactly as directed, otherwise it won't work. Make sure close contacts (such as family and partner) are treated too. The itch can take a few weeks to go away. Don't make the mistake of thinking the treatment hasn't worked –

if you keep putting on the lotion, you'll just irritate the skin more.

Virus This is discussed in the 'Rash' section (p. 117). Some viruses – especially chickenpox – can result in rashes which are quite itchy.

Urticaria Also known as hives or nettle rash. It's usually caused by an allergy to something you've eaten (like nuts, shellfish, or strawberries) or to a medicine (such as an antibiotic). It can also be brought on by viruses and some other rare illnesses. Another type of urticaria, which can keep coming back, can be caused by the skin being irritated by pressure or contact with water.

Treatment Use calamine lotion and antihistamine tablets (like you'd use for hay fever – available from the chemist). If it turns out to be an allergy, avoid the offending food or medicine in the future.

Fungal infections Athlete's foot is an infection caused by a fungus. Similar infections can occur on other areas of the skin, especially where it's moist, such as the armpit or groin (known as 'crutch rot').

Treatment Keep the areas clean and dry and get an antifungal cream from the chemist.

Prickly heat This rash, which can be extremely itchy, appears on areas exposed to the sun. The cause is unknown, but it tends to keep coming back for a few years whenever you go out in the sun in the summer, before it eventually fizzles out.

Treatment The usual calamine lotion and antihistamine tablet routine may help. Stay out of the sun as much as possible, keep cool, and wash the skin regularly.

Psoriasis This is explained, and its treatment outlined, in the 'Rash' section. It can sometimes cause itching.

Other less common causes These include other skin diseases (like lichen planus – see the 'Rash' section, p. 117); certain illnesses (such as diabetes and kidney disease) which can make the skin itch without a rash; psychological problems (stress can set up a vicious cycle of scratching the skin, causing irritation, leading to itching, resulting in further irritation); and the side-effects of medication.

Treatment If you think you have one of these problems, discuss it with your GP.

Knee pain

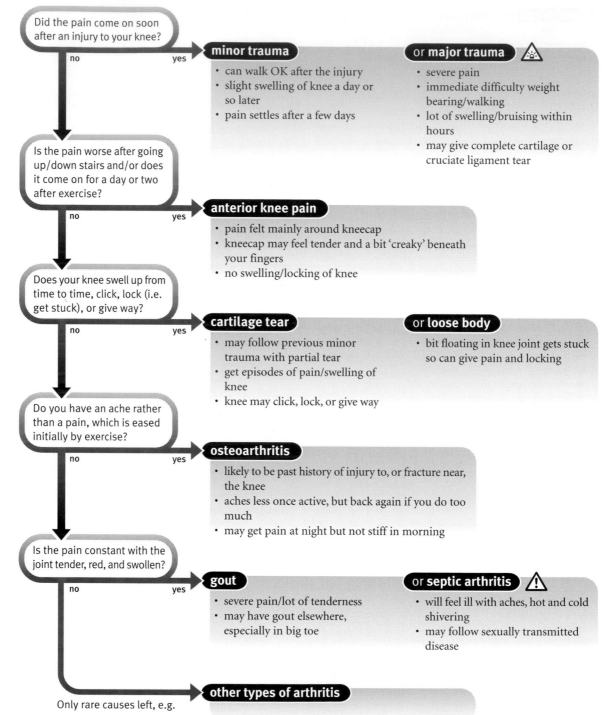

Did the pain come on soon after an injury to your knee?

no — yes →

minor trauma
- can walk OK after the injury
- slight swelling of knee a day or so later
- pain settles after a few days

or major trauma
- severe pain
- immediate difficulty weight bearing/walking
- lot of swelling/bruising within hours
- may give complete cartilage or cruciate ligament tear

Is the pain worse after going up/down stairs and/or does it come on for a day or two after exercise?

no — yes →

anterior knee pain
- pain felt mainly around kneecap
- kneecap may feel tender and a bit 'creaky' beneath your fingers
- no swelling/locking of knee

Does your knee swell up from time to time, click, lock (i.e. get stuck), or give way?

no — yes →

cartilage tear
- may follow previous minor trauma with partial tear
- get episodes of pain/swelling of knee
- knee may click, lock, or give way

or loose body
- bit floating in knee joint gets stuck so can give pain and locking

Do you have an ache rather than a pain, which is eased initially by exercise?

no — yes →

osteoarthritis
- likely to be past history of injury to, or fracture near, the knee
- aches less once active, but back again if you do too much
- may get pain at night but not stiff in morning

Is the pain constant with the joint tender, red, and swollen?

no — yes →

gout
- severe pain/lot of tenderness
- may have gout elsewhere, especially in big toe

or septic arthritis
- will feel ill with aches, hot and cold shivering
- may follow sexually transmitted disease

other types of arthritis

Only rare causes left, e.g.

Minor trauma A mild bump or twist of the knee can cause bruising or a sprain of a ligament (the tough cords holding the knees together). Sometimes, after an injury, the lining of the joint gets inflamed and leaks some fluid, causing slight swelling of the knee a day or so afterwards.

Treatment Remember 'RICE', especially if the knee swells a little: Rest, Ice, Compression, and Elevation. So you should rest the knee for a day or two (elevated on a stool), put an ice-pack on it (like a bag of frozen peas wrapped in a flannel), and use a firm bandage. After a couple of days, the pain should settle – a painkiller may help too (particularly an anti-inflammatory like ibuprofen, which is available from the chemist). Once things are improving, keep the knee strong with quadriceps exercises – the quadriceps are the muscles of the thigh and you can exercise them by putting a weight on your feet and repeatedly straightening out your legs. When you feel confident, get back to your normal activities, including sport – but break yourself back in gently and don't forget to warm up. If you keep getting trouble, see your GP: he might suggest some further treatment such as physiotherapy.

Anterior knee pain This simply means repeated pain in the front of the knee. It's usually caused by a roughening of the underneath of the knee cap or by the thigh muscles inflaming the areas of bone they pull on.

Treatment This usually goes away on its own, although it can take months. If you do a lot of running, try more gentle exercise (like swimming) for a while before gradually getting back into your normal routine. Avoid forcibly bending the knees too much – so keep squatting or kneeling to a minimum. And if you do a lot of cycling, make sure your saddle is high enough to make your legs straighten out when you pedal. Quadriceps exercises and anti-inflammatory pills (as above) may help.

Torn cartilage The cartilage is the knee's shock absorber – it can be torn by a twisting injury.

Treatment A very minor tear may settle with the advice given above for minor trauma. Otherwise, see your GP, who is likely to refer you to an orthopaedic surgeon (a bone specialist).

Osteoarthritis When your knee cartilage gradually wears down, the bones tend to grind over each other, causing a repeated ache – this is osteoarthritis. It's particularly common if you are overweight, have had a serious injury or operation to your knee, or if your knees have suffered through work or sport.

Treatment Painkillers, anti-inflammatories, and quads exercises, as already outlined, are helpful. If you're overweight, try to slim down. Continue exercising, as this keeps the joints supple and the muscles strong – but gentle exercise, like swimming, is much better than anything which jars, such as jogging. You may find that wearing spongy soles, or putting a thick sponge insole into your shoes, acts as a shock absorber, relieving the pressure on your knees. If you're getting nowhere, talk to your GP – but don't expect an X-ray, as this doesn't usually help much. Surgery can cure very arthritic knees, but this is usually reserved for the elderly who are badly disabled by the problem.

Loose body A flake of bone or cartilage can float around in the joint. These 'loose bodies' are often the result of a previous injury.

Treatment This is a job for an orthopaedic specialist if the symptoms are a real nuisance – so speak to your GP, who will probably arrange an appointment for you.

Major trauma A serious knee injury – for example in a road accident, skiing, or on the football pitch – can cause a broken bone or a complete tear of a large ligament (such as the 'ruptured cruciate' – a tear of the main ligaments of the knee). The pain is obviously severe and is usually quickly followed – within an hour or so – by dramatic swelling.

Treatment Go straight to casualty.

(**Gout**) This is covered in the 'Pain in the ankle, foot, or toe' section (p. 97). The knee is the second commonest site for this to happen, after the big toe.

(**Septic arthritis**) This is an infection caused by a germ entering the joint. It's sometimes caused by an infected wound, or, very occasionally, by a sexually transmitted bug entering the bloodstream and ending up in the joint.

Treatment See your GP asap: he is likely to admit you to hospital for powerful antibiotic treatment.

(**Other forms of arthritis**) There are a number of types of joint diseases which can affect the knee, but they are all quite unusual. One type which tends to affect men is Reiter's syndrome, which sometimes comes on after a bout of diarrhoea or a sexually transmitted disease; it can cause skin and eye trouble too. Rheumatoid arthritis can also first show itself through a painful, swollen knee.

Treatment If you think you have this type of problem, see your GP – if he agrees, you're likely to be referred to a joint specialist.

Loss of consciousness

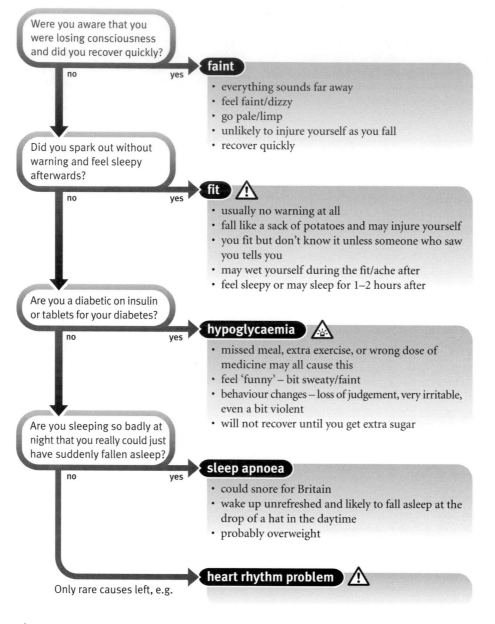

Were you aware that you were losing consciousness and did you recover quickly?

no   yes

faint
- everything sounds far away
- feel faint/dizzy
- go pale/limp
- unlikely to injure yourself as you fall
- recover quickly

Did you spark out without warning and feel sleepy afterwards?

no   yes

fit ⚠
- usually no warning at all
- fall like a sack of potatoes and may injure yourself
- you fit but don't know it unless someone who saw you tells you
- may wet yourself during the fit/ache after
- feel sleepy or may sleep for 1–2 hours after

Are you a diabetic on insulin or tablets for your diabetes?

no   yes

hypoglycaemia ⚠
- missed meal, extra exercise, or wrong dose of medicine may all cause this
- feel 'funny' – bit sweaty/faint
- behaviour changes – loss of judgement, very irritable, even a bit violent
- will not recover until you get extra sugar

Are you sleeping so badly at night that you really could just have suddenly fallen asleep?

no   yes

sleep apnoea
- could snore for Britain
- wake up unrefreshed and likely to fall asleep at the drop of a hat in the daytime
- probably overweight

heart rhythm problem ⚠

Only rare causes left, e.g.

⚠ Anyone who is generally ill and loses consciousness, or who is knocked out after a head injury, should be taken straight to hospital.

Remember: ⚠ means see your GP sharpish; ⚠ means an urgent hospital job

A faint If not enough blood is getting to your brain, you'll pass out – this is nature's way of solving the problem, because you end up horizontal so that your blood isn't having to go uphill anymore to your oxygen-starved brain. A variety of things can trigger a faint. The most typical is standing for a long time somewhere hot and stuffy: normally, your leg movements pump blood back into the circulation, but if you've been standing still for a while, particularly anywhere hot, your blood will 'pool' in your legs, causing a faint. Jumping up quickly out of a hot bath can have the same effect. Other causes include a severe spasm of coughing (which prevents the blood getting to the brain) and sudden fear or pain (which slow the heart rate). Being a bit run down – such as when you have the flu – can also make you more likely to faint. Some people just seem prone to faints and get a number of attacks, but this is almost never caused by any serious disease. Certain medications (such as some blood pressure pills and antidepressants) can also cause faints or near-faints.

Treatment The treatment of someone who is fainting is quite simple – catch him, if you're quick enough, so he doesn't injure himself, then gently lay him down. Raise his feet about 30 degrees in the air, as this will help drain blood back to his brain so that he should recover in a few seconds. If you feel as though you're going to faint, lie down as soon as you can; if this is impossible, sit down with your head between your knees until the feeling has passed. People who are prone to fainting can help prevent attacks by avoiding trigger situations and pumping their calf muscles (by moving their feet up and down as if using an invisible accelerator) if they've been standing still for a while. If you're on prescribed treatment which you think might be causing or aggravating the problem, speak to your GP.

A fit The easiest way to understand a fit is to imagine that the various nerve connections in the brain are like a complex system of electrical wires. A short circuit in this system can result in a variety of types of fit. The most well known is the 'grand mal fit' but there are many other sorts, and some of them can be quite subtle. What causes fits is unknown, although the problem sometimes runs in families. There are a number of things which can trigger fits, including extreme tiredness, an alcoholic binge, flashing lights and, in a known epileptic, forgetting to take your tablets.

Treatment If you think you've had a fit – or someone who was with you at the time reckons that was what happened – make an appointment to see your GP. Try to take someone who can give an eyewitness account, as you'll only be aware of the events leading up to, and immediately after, passing out. Your GP will refer you to a neurologist (a nervous system specialist) for further tests. You're unlikely immediately to be labelled as 'epileptic' as many people suffer just one fit and never have another. If you do get further fits though, you're likely to be told you have epilepsy and you'll be put on treatment to try to keep future fits to a minimum. Remember to inform the DVLC and your car insurers if you develop this problem – you may be banned from driving for a year or more, depending on the circumstances.

Hypoglycaemia This means a low blood sugar level, which effectively starves the brain of energy. If this is the cause of your loss of consciousness, you either have some very rare illness or you're a diabetic. Diabetics on treatment are very prone to this problem, usually because of a missed meal, an unusual amount of exercise, or incorrect doses of diabetic tablets or insulin.

Treatment You need sugar asap. If you're just about conscious enough to swallow then hopefully someone will be forcing a sweet drink down you. But if not, you'll be carted off to hospital for treatment. When you've recovered, try to figure out why it happened. If your sugars have been running low for a while, it may be that your diabetes treatment needs altering. Discuss this with your GP or the local diabetic nurse if you're not confident in making any changes yourself.

Sleep apnoea Loads of people snore badly at night. In a few, the snoring can actually make the breathing stop from time to time. This is sleep apnoea. You won't be aware of this, but your partner will, because she'll be lying awake at night wondering if you've just gasped your last. This problem tends to disturb your sleep and can make you so tired that you tend to drop off ridiculously easily during the day – for example, during a meal or while driving.

Treatment If you're overweight, slim down and avoid alcoholic nightcaps. But if this doesn't sort it out, see your GP, and take your partner with you so she can give him an ear-witness account. You're likely to be referred to an Ear, Nose, and Throat ('ENT') specialist if it's causing real problems.

Rare medical causes There are a few small print causes of loss of consciousness such as heart rhythm or valve problems. They are all very unusual and are likely to produce a variety of other symptoms to give the game away.

Treatment If your GP suspects a rare cause like this, he'll refer you to a specialist for tests.

Loss of sex drive

NB Don't confuse this with difficulties getting an erection; if your problem is not that you've gone off sex, but that you can't get an erection, see the 'Impotence' section.

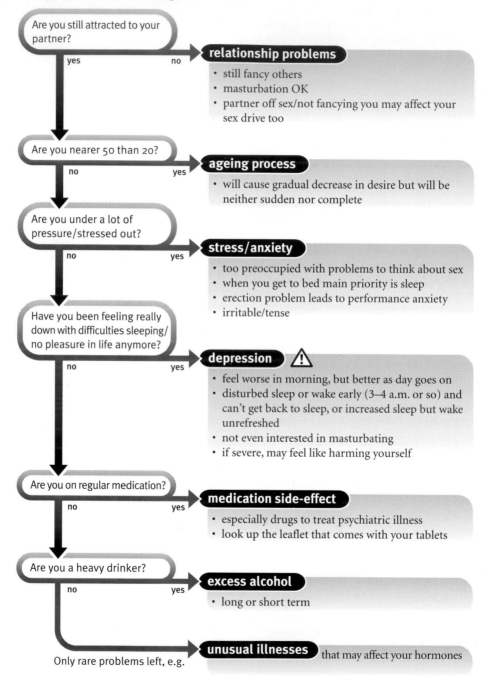

Are you still attracted to your partner?
yes / no

relationship problems
- still fancy others
- masturbation OK
- partner off sex/not fancying you may affect your sex drive too

Are you nearer 50 than 20?
no / yes

ageing process
- will cause gradual decrease in desire but will be neither sudden nor complete

Are you under a lot of pressure/stressed out?
no / yes

stress/anxiety
- too preoccupied with problems to think about sex
- when you get to bed main priority is sleep
- erection problem leads to performance anxiety
- irritable/tense

Have you been feeling really down with difficulties sleeping/ no pleasure in life anymore?
no / yes

depression ⚠
- feel worse in morning, but better as day goes on
- disturbed sleep or wake early (3–4 a.m. or so) and can't get back to sleep, or increased sleep but wake unrefreshed
- not even interested in masturbating
- if severe, may feel like harming yourself

Are you on regular medication?
no / yes

medication side-effect
- especially drugs to treat psychiatric illness
- look up the leaflet that comes with your tablets

Are you a heavy drinker?
no / yes

excess alcohol
- long or short term

unusual illnesses that may affect your hormones

Only rare problems left, e.g.

Stress/anxiety You may simply be too worried about a whole load of problems and stresses to have time to think about sex. And then, as the saying goes, if you don't use it, you lose it – you can fall into the habit of not having sex, and this develops into a lack of interest. Anxiety can affect your sex drive in other ways. For example, you may be worried about getting (or not getting) your partner pregnant, or you might be concerned that you're not performing well in bed. Worries like this – and fear of failure in particular – can end up turning you off sex, because this is a way of avoiding the situation.

Treatment If you're generally feeling tense, look at the advice in the 'Lifestyle/stress' part of the 'Feeling tense' section (p. 59). Try to discuss the situation with your partner, especially if 'performance anxiety' is a large part of the problem. She's bound to have noticed that you've gone off sex, and will probably be worried about the situation too, so it's best to get it out in the open. If the problem doesn't improve, consider seeing your GP – and try to get your partner to go with you. Your GP himself may be able to help, or he may refer you to a psychosexual counsellor (an expert in talking through these problems who can try to help you solve them).

Relationship problems It's not surprising that if you're having constant rows with your partner, or you've simply gone off each other, then your sex life will suffer. Unless the stress is really getting to you, you'll probably still have some sex drive – it just won't be directed towards your partner.

Treatment There's obviously no magic answer to this one other than to try to sort out the problem with your partner.

Depression Your sex drive is one of many areas that depression can affect. It is explained further, and its treatment outlined, in the 'Feeling down' section (p. 57).

Excess alcohol In the short term, after a binge, you may simply be too pissed to care about sex. In the long run, if you booze too much, you can end up with liver damage. This, in turn, alters your hormone levels – including the male sex hormone 'testosterone'. As your testosterone levels drop, so does your sex drive.

Treatment If you're drinking enough to harm your liver, you're in serious trouble and need to see your GP for a check-up and advice. But it's unlikely that alcoholic liver disease will come to light because you've lost your sex drive – it'll usually show itself with other symptoms.

Ageing Testosterone levels gradually fall after you reach your thirties, but, even in old age, most men have enough testosterone circulating to have a reasonable sex drive.

Treatment A mild fall in sex drive is usually regarded as quite normal as men get older, and doesn't usually cause a problem. If your sex drive isn't what you think it should be, it's highly unlikely that the cause is an age-related lack of testosterone. Although testosterone levels can, very rarely, be abnormally low, this is usually caused by unusual illnesses (see below) rather than just age. Although there have been suggestions that men go through a 'male menopause', most doctors believe that this is not the case and view treatments like testosterone tablets or injections as very controversial – so most won't prescribe them.

Medication side-effect Rarely, prescribed medication can lower sex drive – for example, it can occur with some drugs used to treat psychiatric conditions. It's always difficult to know if the problem is an effect of the drug or an effect of the illness the drug is being used to treat.

Treatment If you're on medication which you think could be affecting your sex life, speak to your GP.

Rare medical problems Various unusual illnesses, particularly those which affect hormones, can lower your sex drive.

Treatment It's highly unlikely that you'll have any of these medical rarities. If you're concerned, see your GP, who will check out the problem.

Lumps in the back passage

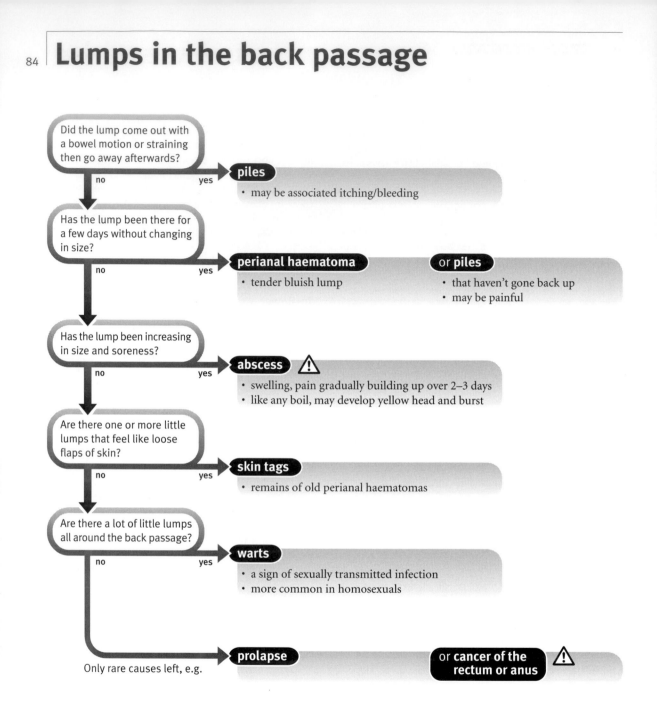

Did the lump come out with a bowel motion or straining then go away afterwards?

no / yes → **piles**
- may be associated itching/bleeding

Has the lump been there for a few days without changing in size?

no / yes → **perianal haematoma**
- tender bluish lump

or piles
- that haven't gone back up
- may be painful

Has the lump been increasing in size and soreness?

no / yes → **abscess** ⚠
- swelling, pain gradually building up over 2–3 days
- like any boil, may develop yellow head and burst

Are there one or more little lumps that feel like loose flaps of skin?

no / yes → **skin tags**
- remains of old perianal haematomas

Are there a lot of little lumps all around the back passage?

no / yes → **warts**
- a sign of sexually transmitted infection
- more common in homosexuals

Only rare causes left, e.g. → **prolapse**

or cancer of the rectum or anus ⚠

Remember: ⚠ means see your GP sharpish; ⚠ means an urgent hospital job

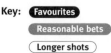
Perianal haematoma This is explained in the 'Pain in the bottom' section (p. 99), which also outlines the treatment.

Piles These are varicose veins (swollen blood vessels) in the back passage. They are usually caused by constipation making you strain when you go to the toilet – this forces blood into the veins. As the veins get bigger, they develop into lumps which poke out of your bottom when you sit on the toilet. They may go back up inside on their own, or you may have to push them up with your finger. Sometimes, they stay out all the time; if they get throttled ('strangulated') by the ring-muscle of your back passage, they get very painful (see the 'Prolapsed piles' part of the 'Pain in the bottom' section, p. 99). They can also bleed if the veins burst (see the 'Bleeding from the back passage' section, p. 27).

Treatment This is fully explained in the 'Bleeding from the back passage' section (p. 27).

Skin tags These are souvenirs of previous perianal haematomas (see above). The blood inside these lumps slowly dissolves away, but, because it has stretched the skin around the back passage, you tend be left with a small, loose flap of skin – these are skin tags.

Treatment Skin tags are totally harmless, usually cause no problem whatsoever, and should simply be left alone.

Abscess This is explained, and the treatment discussed, in the 'Pain in the bottom' section (p. 99). The pain will usually appear before you can actually feel a lump.

Warts These are caused by a virus and are usually passed on sexually – they are more likely to occur around the back passage in homosexuals. Their size varies from tiny pimples to fleshy lumps.

Treatment Your best bet is to go to a 'special clinic' (known under various other names such as 'department of genitourinary medicine', 'sexually transmitted disease clinic', or 'clap clinic'). Most hospitals have these clinics and you don't usually need a letter from your doctor to get an appointment – just ring up and find out when they can see you. They have a number of different treatments which can be used to get rid of the warts (such as special paints or freezing) and they can also check you out for any other sexually transmitted germs. This is important – if you have warts of this sort, you have about a one-in-four chance of some other infection which you wouldn't otherwise have known about. If you are a homosexual, the clinic will also be able to give you advice about avoiding getting more warts in future (like getting your partner to wear an appropriate condom) and information on safe sex in general, should you need it.

Other rare causes These include prolapses and cancer of the back passage. A prolapse means something hanging down – in this case, the lining of your back passage. This is nearly always caused by severe straining because of constipation and is very unusual in the under 50s. Thankfully, cancer of the back passage is also very rare.

Treatment To stop a prolapse getting any worse, sort out your constipation. This means high-fibre foods, plenty of fluids, and more physical exercise. If possible, only use laxatives from the chemist if you're desperate, and just for a week or two. A prolapse in itself isn't harmful, but may be uncomfortable and can irritate or bleed. The only cure is surgery, so discuss the situation with your GP if it's becoming a real problem. If you're worried you might have cancer, then obviously it's a GP job – but you're much more likely to get reassurance or a harmless diagnosis like piles than some bad news and an urgent appointment with a bottom specialist.

Mouth ulcers

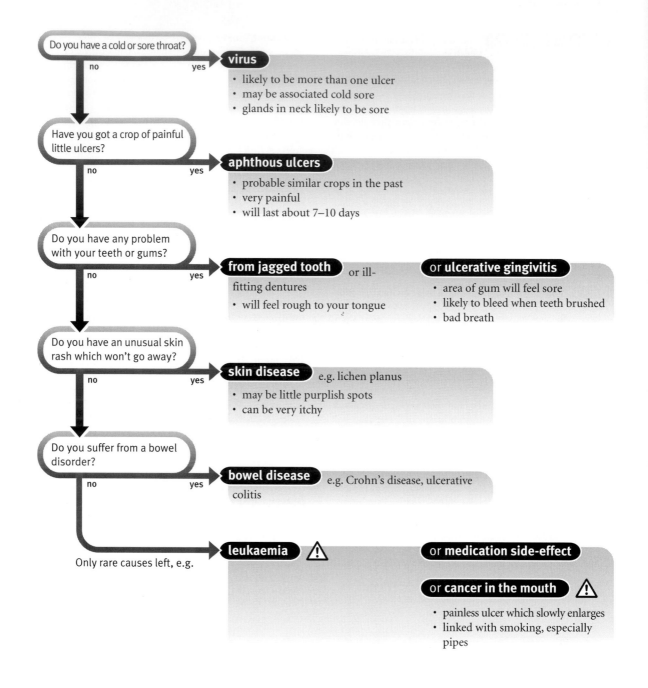

Do you have a cold or sore throat?
no / yes

virus
- likely to be more than one ulcer
- may be associated cold sore
- glands in neck likely to be sore

Have you got a crop of painful little ulcers?
no / yes

aphthous ulcers
- probable similar crops in the past
- very painful
- will last about 7–10 days

Do you have any problem with your teeth or gums?
no / yes

from jagged tooth or ill-fitting dentures
- will feel rough to your tongue

or ulcerative gingivitis
- area of gum will feel sore
- likely to bleed when teeth brushed
- bad breath

Do you have an unusual skin rash which won't go away?
no / yes

skin disease e.g. lichen planus
- may be little purplish spots
- can be very itchy

Do you suffer from a bowel disorder?
no / yes

bowel disease e.g. Crohn's disease, ulcerative colitis

Only rare causes left, e.g.

leukaemia ⚠

or medication side-effect

or cancer in the mouth ⚠
- painless ulcer which slowly enlarges
- linked with smoking, especially pipes

Remember: ⚠ means see your GP sharpish; ⚠ means an urgent hospital job

Aphthous ulcers These are the common mouth ulcers which many people get at times. They are usually very small and may appear in clusters; sometimes, larger single ulcers develop and can take longer to heal. No one knows what causes them, although they sometimes run in families.

Treatment Small ulcers go away on their own in a few days; larger ones can take longer. The chemist will sell you various gels or pastes which may help. As the cause is unknown, there's no real way you can prevent them. It has been suggested that they are a sign of vitamin deficiency, but, in fact, this is hardly ever the case, so vitamin pills almost certainly won't help.

Virus Virus-type germs can cause mouth ulcers among their more familiar symptoms, such as sore throat and fever. For example, a bad attack of the cold sore virus can cause ulcers inside the lips and on the tongue and gums; another virus is known as 'Hand, foot, and mouth' because it causes spots on the hands and feet, and ulcers in the mouth (it has nothing to do with the Foot and Mouth Disease of cows).

Treatment As with most viruses, the only treatment is to wait for the body to fight it off – this normally takes seven to ten days. In the meantime, drink plenty of fluids and take painkillers if necessary.

Trauma from a jagged tooth The sharp edge of a tooth can wear away the surface of the nearby tongue or inner cheek, resulting in an ulcer.

Treatment The ulcer will only clear if the tooth problem is sorted out – so see a dentist.

Ulcerative gingivitis This is an infection of the gums caused by a germ. It is usually linked to neglect of the teeth and gums.

Treatment Another dentist job. Antibiotics will clear the infection, but to prevent future problems the dentist will need to give you a check-up, and you'll have to get working with the brush and floss. Smoking tends to aggravate it too.

Skin disease Some fairly unusual skin diseases can affect the mouth, resulting in ulcers. Occasionally, a disease of this sort causing ulcers leaves the rest of your skin alone, so there may be no skin rashes or blisters to give the game away.

Treatment Discuss the problem with your GP. If you do have skin rashes elsewhere he may be able to piece it all together and treat you, or he may need to refer you to a dermatologist (a skin specialist). Sometimes a biopsy (the removal of a tiny bit of the skin of the mouth where there's an ulcer) is needed to work out exactly what's going on – you will be referred to a hospital specialist for this.

Bowel disease Some diseases of the gut, such as ulcerative colitis and Crohn's disease (see the 'Diarrhoea' section, p. 47), can cause repeated attacks of mouth ulcers.

Treatment The ulcers themselves are treated in much the same way as aphthous ulcers (see above). For treatment of bowel disease, see the 'Diarrhoea' section (p. 47).

Blood disorder Serious blood diseases, like leukaemia, can very rarely show themselves through severe and persistent mouth ulcers, although there are usually lots of other symptoms too. The side-effects of some prescribed drugs (such as anti-thyroid and rheumatoid arthritis treatments) can cause blood problems, which also lead to mouth ulcers. If you're on one of these drugs, which is unlikely, you'll probably have been told to look out for this particular problem and report it to your doctor.

Treatment See your GP urgently for a blood test.

Cancer Cancer of the lip, tongue, or mouth may start with a painless ulcer which slowly enlarges. This problem is very rare in the under 45s and may be linked with smoking and excess alcohol.

Treatment Any unexplained mouth ulcer which gets larger over weeks needs checking by your GP. If he's at all concerned, he'll refer you to a specialist for a biopsy (see above).

Multiple joint pains

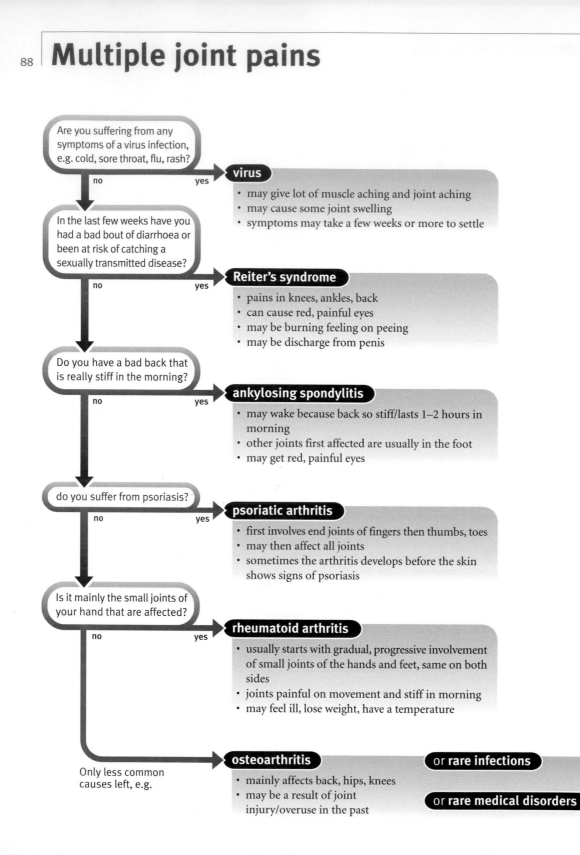

Are you suffering from any symptoms of a virus infection, e.g. cold, sore throat, flu, rash?

no / **yes**

virus
- may give lot of muscle aching and joint aching
- may cause some joint swelling
- symptoms may take a few weeks or more to settle

In the last few weeks have you had a bad bout of diarrhoea or been at risk of catching a sexually transmitted disease?

no / **yes**

Reiter's syndrome
- pains in knees, ankles, back
- can cause red, painful eyes
- may be burning feeling on peeing
- may be discharge from penis

Do you have a bad back that is really stiff in the morning?

no / **yes**

ankylosing spondylitis
- may wake because back so stiff/lasts 1–2 hours in morning
- other joints first affected are usually in the foot
- may get red, painful eyes

do you suffer from psoriasis?

no / **yes**

psoriatic arthritis
- first involves end joints of fingers then thumbs, toes
- may then affect all joints
- sometimes the arthritis develops before the skin shows signs of psoriasis

Is it mainly the small joints of your hand that are affected?

no / **yes**

rheumatoid arthritis
- usually starts with gradual, progressive involvement of small joints of the hands and feet, same on both sides
- joints painful on movement and stiff in morning
- may feel ill, lose weight, have a temperature

Only less common causes left, e.g.

osteoarthritis
- mainly affects back, hips, knees
- may be a result of joint injury/overuse in the past

or rare infections

or rare medical disorders

Virus A lot of viruses can result in joint aches, or even joint swellings, along with all the other symptoms they cause. Examples include flu, hepatitis, glandular fever, and German measles.

Treatment There is no magic cure for viruses – they just have to work their way out of the system. Joint pains can sometimes take a few weeks to settle down, and can be helped by anti-inflammatory drugs (such as ibuprofen – available from the chemist). You'll need to see your GP to check that the cause is a virus and for him to give you further advice depending on the particular germ you've been infected with.

Reiter's syndrome This is an illness caused either by a sexually transmitted germ or by certain bugs which lead to diarrhoea. It is one of the commonest types of arthritis in young men and usually affects the knees, ankles, or back. It can also cause eye and skin problems.

Treatment This illness usually clears up after about three months, although it can come back again. You'll probably end up seeing a rheumatologist (a joint specialist) who will keep an eye on you and treat you with anti-inflammatory drugs. If the problem was triggered by a sexually transmitted germ, you'll probably also be given antibiotics – this is likely to be arranged by another specialist at the clinic for sexually transmitted diseases.

Ankylosing spondylitis This form of arthritis affects blokes under the age of 30, causing low back pain and stiffness, pain in the joints of the rib cage and, sometimes, pain and swelling in other joints. The cause is unknown, though it sometimes runs in families.

Treatment This is another job for the rheumatologist. Apart from prescribing you various treatments, your specialist will advise you about keeping active and supple: it's very important to take regular exercise, such as swimming, and to improve your posture.

Psoriatic arthritis A few people who suffer with psoriasis – a common skin condition causing a scaly rash – also get a particular type of arthritis. This usually affects the hands, although other joints can also cause trouble.

Treatment See your GP. If your arthritis isn't too bad, he may just treat you with anti-inflammatory drugs. But if they don't work, or your problem is severe, you'll be referred to the rheumatologist, who may need to use more powerful drugs to stop your joints getting too damaged.

Rheumatoid arthritis This type of arthritis usually starts between the ages of 30 and 50, initially affecting the hands, wrists, and feet. The exact cause is unknown.

Treatment If your GP thinks you may have this problem, he'll refer you to a rheumatologist. Rheumatoid arthritis can cause a lot of damage to your joints and to other parts of your body, so your specialist will give you advice about looking after your joints and will treat you with anti-inflammatory drugs or more powerful treatments to keep the arthritis at bay.

Osteoarthritis This is 'wear and tear' type arthritis. It's common in older age groups – about two-thirds of men aged over 50 have signs of osteoarthritis if their joints are X-rayed. But it's much less common in younger blokes. It can occur if you've made your joints suffer in the past (such as through playing loads of footy) or if you've had other joint problems (especially knee cartilage surgery) – in these situations, the knees and hips are the likeliest to have problems.

Treatment The main points in treating osteoarthritis can be found in the 'Osteoarthritis' part of the 'Knee pain' section.

Rare infections Some pretty unusual infections can cause joint pains among their various other symptoms. These include gonorrhoea (a sexually transmitted germ which usually also results in a discharge from the penis and burning on peeing), Lyme disease (caused by a tick bite), and brucellosis (a germ picked up from cattle, so a hazard to vets, abattoir workers, and so on).

Treatment See your GP – and tell him why you think you might have one of these rarities.

Other rare medical disorders There are a load of rare types of arthritis and small print illnesses which can cause joint pains.

Treatment The chances are you haven't got any of them. If you're concerned, see your GP, who will run any necessary tests.

Nail problems

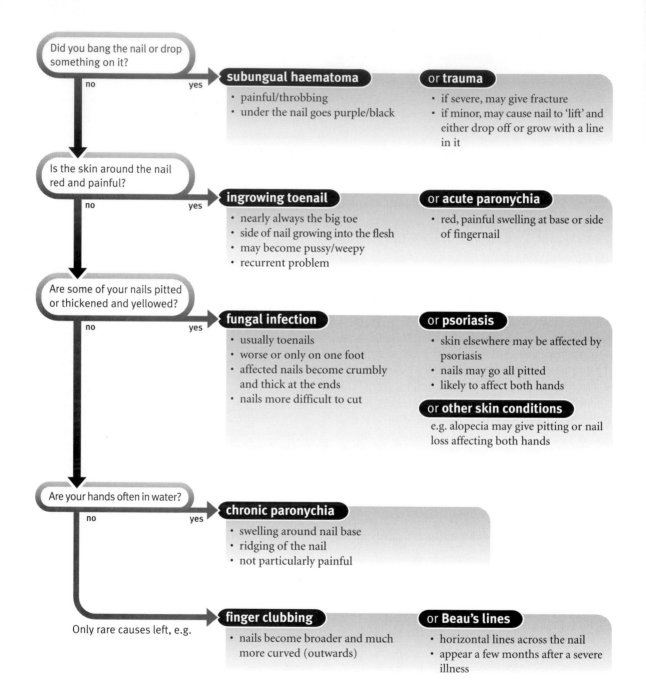

Did you bang the nail or drop something on it?
no / yes

subungual haematoma
- painful/throbbing
- under the nail goes purple/black

or trauma
- if severe, may give fracture
- if minor, may cause nail to 'lift' and either drop off or grow with a line in it

Is the skin around the nail red and painful?
no / yes

ingrowing toenail
- nearly always the big toe
- side of nail growing into the flesh
- may become pussy/weepy
- recurrent problem

or acute paronychia
- red, painful swelling at base or side of fingernail

Are some of your nails pitted or thickened and yellowed?
no / yes

fungal infection
- usually toenails
- worse or only on one foot
- affected nails become crumbly and thick at the ends
- nails more difficult to cut

or psoriasis
- skin elsewhere may be affected by psoriasis
- nails may go all pitted
- likely to affect both hands

or other skin conditions
e.g. alopecia may give pitting or nail loss affecting both hands

Are your hands often in water?
no / yes

chronic paronychia
- swelling around nail base
- ridging of the nail
- not particularly painful

Only rare causes left, e.g.

finger clubbing
- nails become broader and much more curved (outwards)

or Beau's lines
- horizontal lines across the nail
- appear a few months after a severe illness

Subungual haematoma Blood under the nail. This happens after an injury – typically after accidentally thwacking the nail with a hammer. Because the blood is under pressure, it hurts like hell.

Treatment If you can bear the pain, it's safe to leave it alone, as the blood will get reabsorbed after a few days. But if it's really throbbing and you're feeling brave, you can try making a hole in the nail. Simply heat up the tip of an unfolded paper clip or a pin until it's red hot. Then place the tip in the centre of your nail and grit your teeth. It will burn a hole through your nail and the blood, under pressure, will suddenly spurt out, giving you instant relief. The only pain you'll feel is when you finally get through the nail and touch the sensitive tissue underneath – this only lasts a second. Don't try this trick if you've really mangled your finger or thumb badly, though – if there's a broken bone, making a hole could introduce infection. Go to casualty instead.

Ingrowing toenail This almost always affects the big toe. The side of the nail grows into the flesh, which becomes swollen and sore. It can also get infected, making it hurt and swell more, and discharge pus.

Treatment Avoid narrow-toed shoes and cut the nail straight across rather than in a curve. An antiseptic cream may cure an early infection, but, if it's very mucky, sore, and swollen, you'll probably need antibiotics. But these only clear the infection, not the ingrowing nail itself. There are a couple of DIY treatments you can try. Cutting a tiny 'V' into the middle of the top of the nail makes it slightly more flexible – this relieves the pressure from the ingrowing edge. Alternatively, using the blunt end of a cocktail stick, wedge a plug of cotton wool soaked in disinfectant under the ingrowing part. Repeat this trick daily and you may be able to cure yourself, although, as the nail grows very slowly, it can take up to three months. If all else fails, your GP can arrange for you to have a minor operation to sort it out.

Acute paronychia An infection caused by a germ getting under the skin at the base of the nail.

Treatment If it's just started, see your GP for some antibiotics. But if it's gone on for a few days and the swelling is very tender and soft, it'll need lancing to let the pus out. This may be a GP or hospital job – give your doc a ring and see what he says.

Trauma A more minor injury can make the nail lift up as it grows out. Alternatively, it might develop a groove or ridge.

Treatment There's nothing you need to do about this. If the nail comes off, don't worry. It'll feel sore for a few days, but a new nail will grow.

Fungal infection A fungus can get into the nail and make it thicken and crumble.

Treatment These infections are difficult to clear, so if it's not bothering you, leave it alone. It might eventually go on its own, or you might just have to clip or file it down occasionally. If it's causing pain or you hate the way it looks, see your GP, as there are anti-fungal tablets available which might cure the problem.

Psoriasis This is explained in the 'Rash' section. Some people with psoriasis find it causes problems with their nails too, including small pits and thickening.

Treatment There is no effective treatment for this problem.

Other skin conditions Skin and nails are closely linked, so various skin problems, like hand eczema and alopecia arcata (see 'Hair loss' section, p. 61), can also damage the nails.

Treatment Again, treatments don't really help at all.

Chronic paronychia If you frequently have your hands in water – maybe you're a barman or you haven't invested in a dishwasher yet – the thin rim of skin at the base of the nail (the cuticle) may disappear. This allows a type of fungus to enter the skin, causing slight swelling around the nail base, and ridging of the nail itself. This is chronic paronychia.

Treatment The cure lies in keeping your hands out of water. If that's impossible, make sure you wear gloves with a cotton liner. An anti-fungal cream (such as clotrimazole, which is available from the chemist) applied to the swollen area may also help, though it may take weeks.

Rare problems Examples include Beau's lines and clubbing. Any severe illness can slow down nail growth. This results in horizontal lines (Beau's lines) appearing across all the nails (especially the fingernails). Usually, these only become noticeable a few months after the illness which has caused them. Various rare conditions (like lung or bowel disease) can affect the way the nails grow, resulting in nails which broaden and curve (in the direction of a claw). The fingertips may grow the same way too. This is known as 'clubbing'.

Treatment No treatment is needed for Beau's lines as they will grow out. If you've had clubbing since childbirth and it's in the family too, then it's a type handed down through the generations and is harmless. But if it's developed recently, see your GP. If he thinks there's a problem, he'll arrange any necessary tests.

Noises in the ear

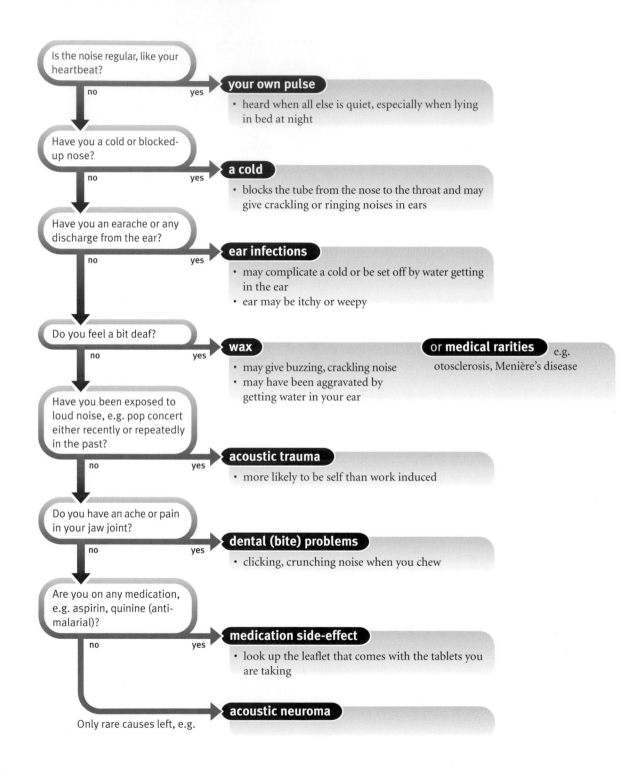

Is the noise regular, like your heartbeat?

no   yes

your own pulse
- heard when all else is quiet, especially when lying in bed at night

Have you a cold or blocked-up nose?

no   yes

a cold
- blocks the tube from the nose to the throat and may give crackling or ringing noises in ears

Have you an earache or any discharge from the ear?

no   yes

ear infections
- may complicate a cold or be set off by water getting in the ear
- ear may be itchy or weepy

Do you feel a bit deaf?

no   yes

wax
- may give buzzing, crackling noise
- may have been aggravated by getting water in your ear

or medical rarities e.g. otosclerosis, Menière's disease

Have you been exposed to loud noise, e.g. pop concert either recently or repeatedly in the past?

no   yes

acoustic trauma
- more likely to be self than work induced

Do you have an ache or pain in your jaw joint?

no   yes

dental (bite) problems
- clicking, crunching noise when you chew

Are you on any medication, e.g. aspirin, quinine (anti-malarial)?

no   yes

medication side-effect
- look up the leaflet that comes with the tablets you are taking

acoustic neuroma

Only rare causes left, e.g.

Noises in the ear

Your own pulse Most of the time, you won't be aware of this – but if everything is quiet (usually at night), you may hear the pulse in your ear. This is most likely to happen if your pulse is harder or faster than usual, such as if you're anxious or have a fever.

Treatment This is normal and so needs no treatment. Turning over on to the other side may get rid of it if it's bothering you when you're lying in bed.

A cold Caused by a virus and inflames the ear, nose, and throat. Catarrh tends to block the inner tubes causing pressure changes in your ears, making them feel as though they want to 'pop'. Pressure on the eardrums produces a sensation of ringing in the ears (tinnitus).

Treatment There is no magic cure for a cold, so there's no point seeing your GP. The symptoms will disappear after a few days. The stuffed-up feeling and noises in the ears may be helped by steam inhalations – put a towel over your head, then put your head over a bowl of hot water and breathe in the steam.

Ear wax This is explained in the section on 'Deafness' (p. 45). Wax can press on the eardrum, causing tinnitus.

Treatment See the section on 'Deafness' (p. 45).

Ear infections There are different types of infections which can affect the ear. Some just cause problems with the ear canal, others go deeper and affect the eardrum and beyond. Some are 'one-offs', others keep coming back, and others stay there constantly until dealt with by your GP or a specialist. They can all cause an ear discharge and this, together with possible damage to the drum and other parts of the ear, can lead to tinnitus.

Treatment A GP job to sort out the type of infection and prescribe you the right treatment – probably either drops or antibiotics. You might have to see an Ear, Nose, and Throat ('ENT') specialist if the infection is difficult to shift or causing a lot of problems. For the future, you can keep problems to a minimum by avoiding cotton buds and keeping water out of your ears – so use ear plugs or a wedge of cotton wool dipped in vaseline when you're swimming or washing your hair.

Acoustic trauma This means damage caused by loud noises. It's normal to feel ringing in the ears after a sudden loud noise, such as an explosion – this usually goes away quickly. Repeated exposure to noise, such as working in a noisy environment without ear protection, or overdoses of heavy metal through earphones, can damage the ear, resulting in long-term tinnitus and deafness.

Treatment It's important to protect the ears from further problems by wearing ear protection at work and cutting down on raucous music through earphones. Unfortunately, tinnitus of this sort cannot be cured. If it's causing you real problems, it's worth talking to your GP. Treatments that can help include masking devices (aids which produce a 'white noise', blocking out the tinnitus), psychological help (to train you how to relax and ignore the noise), and anti-depressants (if the symptom is really getting you down).

Dental problems Dental trouble, especially if it puts the 'bite' of your upper and lower teeth out of line, can inflame the jaw joint (the temporomandibular joint). As a result, you'll notice clicking and crunching sounds, particularly when you chew.

Treatment Bite the bullet and see your dentist.

Medication side-effect Over-the-counter treatments such as aspirin and ibuprofen, and prescribed drugs like quinine (used for cramps and prevention of malaria for travellers abroad), can produce tinnitus as a side-effect – especially if you take more than the recommended dose.

Treatment Stop the offending drug. If you've accidentally or deliberately exceeded the stated dose, get urgent medical help by going straight to casualty.

Medical rarities There are some uncommon illnesses which can cause ringing in the ears. These include Menière's disease (raised pressure of the fluid deep in the ears), oto-sclerosis (seizing up of the tiny bones in the ear), and acoustic neuroma (a growth on the nerve leading away from the ear).

Treatment See your GP. If he's concerned, he'll send you to an ENT specialist for tests and treatment.

Odd behaviour

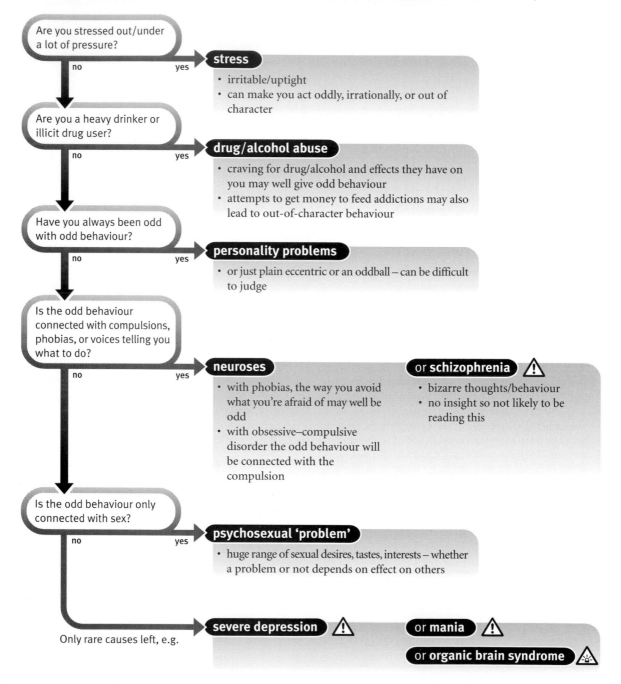

If you are a diabetic, treat odd behaviour as hypoglycaemia until proved otherwise.

NB The problem here is that you may not think your behaviour is odd at all because, in some of the more serious conditions, you lose touch with reality. So hand the book over to your nearest and dearest, and let them sort you out.

Are you stressed out/under a lot of pressure?
no → yes

stress
- irritable/uptight
- can make you act oddly, irrationally, or out of character

Are you a heavy drinker or illicit drug user?
no → yes

drug/alcohol abuse
- craving for drug/alcohol and effects they have on you may well give odd behaviour
- attempts to get money to feed addictions may also lead to out-of-character behaviour

Have you always been odd with odd behaviour?
no → yes

personality problems
- or just plain eccentric or an oddball – can be difficult to judge

Is the odd behaviour connected with compulsions, phobias, or voices telling you what to do?
no → yes

neuroses
- with phobias, the way you avoid what you're afraid of may well be odd
- with obsessive–compulsive disorder the odd behaviour will be connected with the compulsion

or schizophrenia
- bizarre thoughts/behaviour
- no insight so not likely to be reading this

Is the odd behaviour only connected with sex?
no → yes

psychosexual 'problem'
- huge range of sexual desires, tastes, interests – whether a problem or not depends on effect on others

Only rare causes left, e.g.

severe depression

or mania

or organic brain syndrome

Stress Being under pressure all the time – typically because of work, relationship, or money worries – will make you feel constantly uptight. The result is usually a short fuse: it won't take much to make you explode, so you may experience outbursts of anger or you may even get violent. Alternatively, you might get depressed and weepy.

Treatment Look at the 'Feeling tense' (p. 59) or 'Feeling down' (p. 57) section, depending on whether you're feeling uptight or depressed.

Drug and alcohol abuse Mind-expanding drugs will obviously alter your behaviour. Alcohol does the same. Suddenly stopping after long-term use can cause a 'withdrawal syndrome', with cravings, physical symptoms, and odd behaviour. Also, in the long run, being hooked on drugs or booze can change your personality, because you'll lead a chaotic lifestyle and probably end up skint – for example, you may become short tempered, devious, and suspicious of other people.

Treatment Cut down on the drugs and booze – and preferably stop them altogether. If you think you need help, see your GP or contact the local drug or alcohol unit.

Personality problems It's a matter of opinion when a personality crosses the line from being normal to abnormal. But psychiatrists do recognize certain types of personality which, when extreme, can cause problems, either to the individual or to those around him. These include the psychopath (aggressive, often in trouble with the law, antisocial) and the paranoid (oversensitive and suspicious), although there are many others. The cause of these exaggerated personalities is probably a mixture of family traits and a disturbed childhood.

Treatment Personalities can't be changed, so there's no 'cure', but psychologists and psychiatrists can sometimes help people to alter their behaviour – speak to your GP.

Neuroses These are a variety of psychiatric problems which all result in anxiety. They include, among others, phobias and panic attacks. They are explained in more detail, and their treatments discussed, in the 'Feeling tense' section (p. 59).

Schizophrenia This is a serious psychiatric problem causing a pattern of odd symptoms and behaviour (see flow chart). It usually starts in your early 20s and its cause is unknown, although it may result from chemical imbalances in the brain.

Treatment This needs the help of your GP, who, in turn, will probably call in a psychiatrist. You may not realize you're ill; you might even need to be 'forced' to go into hospital under the Mental Health Act (a law which enables doctors to insist that you have treatment even when you don't want it). Medication is usually in the form of tablets and injections. Unfortunately, the problem tends to come back, so you'll need ongoing help and monitoring from your GP, psychiatrist, or a mental health nurse.

Depression This is explained, and its treatment outlined, in the 'Feeling down' section (p. 57). Serious depression can, very occasionally, make you lose touch with reality, develop bizarre, negative thoughts, and behave oddly.

Psychosexual problem There is an astonishing range of odd sexual behaviour (ranging from foot fetishism and bondage through to stealing women's underwear and flashing). What is regarded as 'abnormal' depends on your partner, society, and the law.

Treatment If your psychosexual problem is causing you, or others, problems, speak to your GP. He will probably refer you to a psychosexual counsellor (a 'sexpert') or a psychiatrist.

Mania This is another serious psychiatric problem in which you totally lose touch with reality. It tends to keep coming back and may alternate with attacks of depression. The cause is unknown.

Treatment Much the same as for schizophrenia (see above). Medication can also be used to try to prevent attacks.

Organic brain syndrome This is any physical illness which clouds how the brain works. There are loads of causes. Some are sudden (e.g. a head injury or meningitis) and others are gradual (e.g. a brain tumour or CJD). A few medications can, rarely, have the same effect (e.g. steroids and some blood pressure pills). In diabetics on treatment, a common cause is hypoglycaemia (a low blood sugar) caused, for example, by a missed meal or excess exercise.

Treatment These situations obviously require medical attention – urgently in the case of problems with a sudden onset. If you're a diabetic and you think you're having a 'hypo', get some sugar down you asap.

Pain in the ankle, foot, or toe

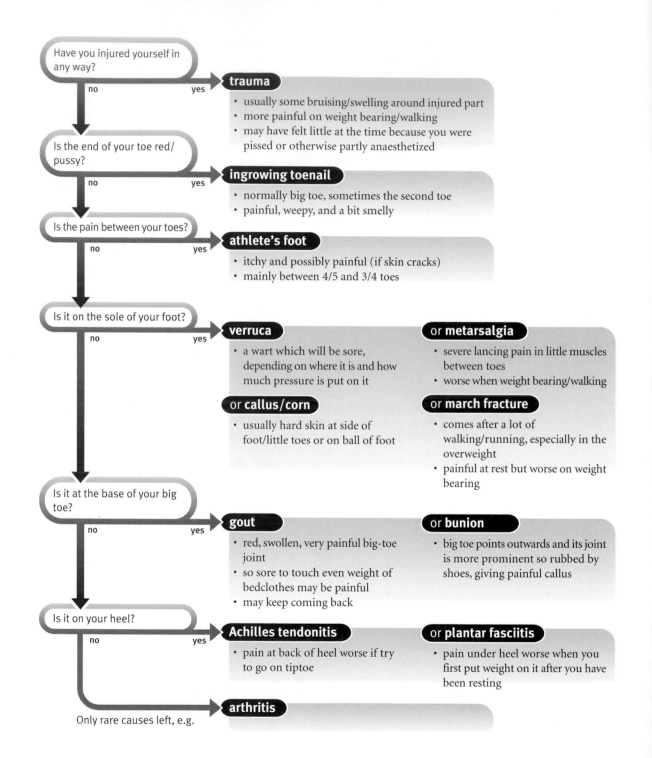

Have you injured yourself in any way? no / yes → **trauma**
- usually some bruising/swelling around injured part
- more painful on weight bearing/walking
- may have felt little at the time because you were pissed or otherwise partly anaesthetized

Is the end of your toe red/pussy? no / yes → **ingrowing toenail**
- normally big toe, sometimes the second toe
- painful, weepy, and a bit smelly

Is the pain between your toes? no / yes → **athlete's foot**
- itchy and possibly painful (if skin cracks)
- mainly between 4/5 and 3/4 toes

Is it on the sole of your foot? no / yes →

verruca
- a wart which will be sore, depending on where it is and how much pressure is put on it

or callus/corn
- usually hard skin at side of foot/little toes or on ball of foot

or metarsalgia
- severe lancing pain in little muscles between toes
- worse when weight bearing/walking

or march fracture
- comes after a lot of walking/running, especially in the overweight
- painful at rest but worse on weight bearing

Is it at the base of your big toe? no / yes →

gout
- red, swollen, very painful big-toe joint
- so sore to touch even weight of bedclothes may be painful
- may keep coming back

or bunion
- big toe points outwards and its joint is more prominent so rubbed by shoes, giving painful callus

Is it on your heel? no / yes →

Achilles tendonitis
- pain at back of heel worse if try to go on tiptoe

or plantar fasciitis
- pain under heel worse when you first put weight on it after you have been resting

→ **arthritis**

Only rare causes left, e.g.

Pain in the ankle, foot, or toe

Trauma For ankle injuries, see the 'Ankle swelling' section. Twisting your ankle can cause other injuries, like a bit of bone being pulled off the outer edge of your foot.

Treatment If you may have broken a bone – a severe injury, a lot of bruising, and swelling or you can't bear weight – you need to go to casualty. Otherwise, if it's really sore, use ice-packs and painkillers and rest the injured part for a day or two.

Athlete's foot This is an infection between the webs of the toes caused by a fungus. It's usually itchy, but it can be sore if it makes the skin crack.

Treatment Keep your feet dry and use an anti-fungal cream from the chemist.

Ingrowing toenail A nail which curves into the skin, making it swollen and sore. It can get infected, in which case it goes red, gets more painful, and leaks pus.

Treatment Avoid narrow-toed shoes and cut the nail straight across rather than in a curve. Try a couple of DIY tricks: wedge a plug of antiseptic-soaked cotton wool under the ingrowing edge each day – this 'persuades' the nail to grow out of the skin, but takes weeks or even months to work. Or you can cut a small 'V' in the middle of the front edge of the nail, as this relieves the pressure on the sides. If it gets infected, you'll need antibiotics from your GP – and if you get problems for months without any signs of improvement, talk to him about a small operation to sort it out.

Verruca This is a wart growing into the sole of the foot.

Treatment It's best to leave it alone as it'll go on its own eventually. If it's a nuisance, soak the foot each evening to soften the skin, then rub the verruca with a pumice stone – keep this up for a few weeks and you may succeed in filing it down to nothing.

Callus/corn This is hard skin caused by friction. It may develop on the sole of the foot or where one toe rubs against another.

Treatment As for a verruca (see above).

Bunion If your big toe starts to point in towards your other toes, its base sticks out and get rubbed by your shoes. This makes the base of the toe inflamed.

Treatment If it's a problem, try pads to relieve the pressure or strapping to straighten the toe (both available from the chemist). If you're desperate, surgery can help.

Gout In your blood there is a chemical called 'uric acid'. In some people, the level of this chemical is high enough for them to develop uric acid crystals, which get stuck in joints (especially the big-toe joint), causing severe inflammation. It may run in families and it's aggravated by being over-weight or boozing too much.

Treatment If it's your first attack, you're bound to see the doc as it's so painful. Rest the toe, and use ice-packs and the anti-inflammatory drug your GP will prescribe. Keep some handy in case you get further attacks. To cut the chances of further problems, shed any excess pounds and don't overdo the alcohol. If you do keep getting attacks, see your GP, as he may prescribe you treatment to try to prevent the problem.

Achilles tendonitis The Achilles tendon is the tough, thick cord connecting your calf to your heel. 'Tendonitis' is inflammation of the tendon – usually the result of overdo-ing exercise or the heel tab of your trainer rubbing on it.

Treatment Rest for a few weeks then gradually start exer-cising again, avoiding trainers with high heel tabs. Anti-inflammatory drugs (available over the counter) may help.

Metatarsalgia This is pain in the ball of the foot. It has a number of causes, including new shoes, too much running, and a trapped nerve.

Treatment Padding under the ball of the foot and anti-inflammatory drugs may help. If the problem persists, see your GP for further advice and treatment.

Plantar fasciitis An inflammation of the sole of the foot (mainly the heel area). Again, this can be caused by new shoes or by doing unusual amounts of walking or running.

Treatment A heel pad and anti-inflammatories may help. Otherwise, you'll probably need a cortisone injection, so see your GP.

March fracture A stress fracture of a bone in the foot – usually caused by excess running on hard surfaces.

Treatment This needs about six weeks' rest, then a gradual return to exercise – preferably with better shoes and on a softer surface.

Arthritis Various types of arthritis can affect the ankles (see the 'Ankle swelling' (p. 19) and 'Multiple joint pains' (p. 89) sections). Osteoarthritis (wear and tear) can affect the big toe.

Treatment For ankle problems, see the sections mentioned above. Big-toe arthritis is usually helped by painkillers and padding.

Pain in the bottom

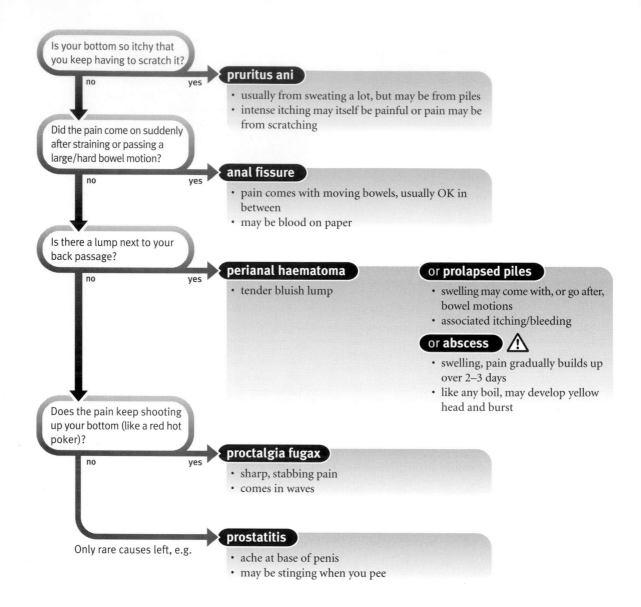

Is your bottom so itchy that you keep having to scratch it?

no — yes →

pruritus ani
- usually from sweating a lot, but may be from piles
- intense itching may itself be painful or pain may be from scratching

Did the pain come on suddenly after straining or passing a large/hard bowel motion?

no — yes →

anal fissure
- pain comes with moving bowels, usually OK in between
- may be blood on paper

Is there a lump next to your back passage?

no — yes →

perianal haematoma
- tender bluish lump

or prolapsed piles
- swelling may come with, or go after, bowel motions
- associated itching/bleeding

or abscess ⚠
- swelling, pain gradually builds up over 2–3 days
- like any boil, may develop yellow head and burst

Does the pain keep shooting up your bottom (like a red hot poker)?

no — yes →

proctalgia fugax
- sharp, stabbing pain
- comes in waves

Only rare causes left, e.g.

prostatitis
- ache at base of penis
- may be stinging when you pee

Remember: ⚠ means see your GP sharpish; ⚠ means an urgent hospital job

Pruritus ani Itching around the tail-end. It can get very sore, especially if you scratch it a lot. There are lots of different things which can cause it in the first place, such as sweating and eczema, but it's the scratching which keeps it going by inflaming the sensitive skin.

Treatment There are two key steps to sorting this out. First, keep the area clean and dry – the easiest way is to use wet-wipes to clean thoroughly each time you open your bowels. Second, stop scratching – it won't have a chance to heal up if you're tearing the skin to pieces. You can also try small amounts of hydrocortisone 1% cream from the chemist twice a day, as this will ease the itching. If all else fails, discuss the problem with your doc, as you may need a 'prescription-only' cream, or some other treatment, to sort it out.

Perianal haematoma A burst blood vessel next to the back passage. The blood leaks into, and stretches, the skin, giving a tender, bluish, cherry-sized lump (technically, a 'haematoma'). It's usually caused by straining when you're constipated, or by a bout of diarrhoea.

Treatment It will go away on its own after five days or so. You'll be left with a tiny soft lump – a 'skin tag' – which is harmless and so can be ignored. Because the haematoma hurts, it's tempting to avoid opening your bowels regularly – but you must, otherwise you'll get constipated, and any straining runs the risk of developing another one straight away. If the pain is agonizing, consider going to casualty, as it's possible to have the lump cut open so that the blood inside can be shelled out, relieving the pressure. On the other hand, you might just want to grit your teeth for a few days. It's certainly worth increasing your fibre intake for the future, to cut down the chance of further problems.

Anal fissure A small tear in the back passage. The causes are the same as for a perianal haematoma (see above).

Treatment This, too, will usually sort itself out, though it may take a week or two. Again, it's important not to let the pain get you constipated – straining or passing huge logs will open up the split again. If possible, have a quick dunk in a bath each time you've opened your bowels, as this will ease the pain and help keep the area clean. You can also try lignocaine gel or ointment (an anaesthetic) from the chemist – rub it into the sore area about half an hour before, and shortly after, going to the toilet. Very occasionally, the fissure won't heal. So if it's going on for weeks without improving, see your GP. You may need to be referred to a specialist for a small operation.

Prolapsed piles Piles are simply varicose veins (swollen blood vessels) in the back passage (see 'Lumps in the back passage' section, p. 85). They aren't usually painful, but if they drop down and poke out of your bottom – in other words, prolapse – they can get sore.

Treatment If they pop back in after you've been to the toilet, they're unlikely to cause you too many problems. Simply avoid getting too constipated (as above). If they stay out all the time, they're more likely to cause pain and bleeding. Any of the heaps of creams available from the chemist will help the soreness, but they're likely to need other treatment – possibly a small operation – so see your GP. Very occasionally, prolapsed piles which stay out can become 'strangulated' – throttled by the muscle of your back passage. This causes severe pain and swelling: next stop, casualty.

Abscess A skin infection which can develop into a large, hot, painful lump.

Treatment An abscess needs, at best, a course of antibiotics and, at worst, a trip to the hospital for lancing. So see the doc – urgently if the lump is large, very painful, and you feel unwell and feverish.

Proctalgia fugax A severe pain in the back passage. The bad news is that no one knows what causes it. The good news is that it's harmless.

Treatment A really tough one. There is no cure and no consistently effective treatment. Some find hot baths useful, others use ice-packs, and some find massage in or around the back passage stops an attack. Otherwise it's a case of either dosing yourself up with a strong painkiller or seeing if your GP might try you on a prescribed treatment – some doctors have found that an ointment usually used to treat angina seems to help proctalgia when applied to the tail-end (just don't ask how they discovered this).

Prostatitis An infection of the prostate gland caused by a germ. This usually enters through the penis and travels up to the gland, which is the size of a walnut and sits just under the bladder. When infected, it can cause a variety of symptoms, including a pain in the bottom.

Treatment See your GP for this one. He'll probably want to examine you – including the notorious finger up the bottom routine – and if this confirms prostatitis, you're probably in for a long course of antibiotics.

Pain in the testicle

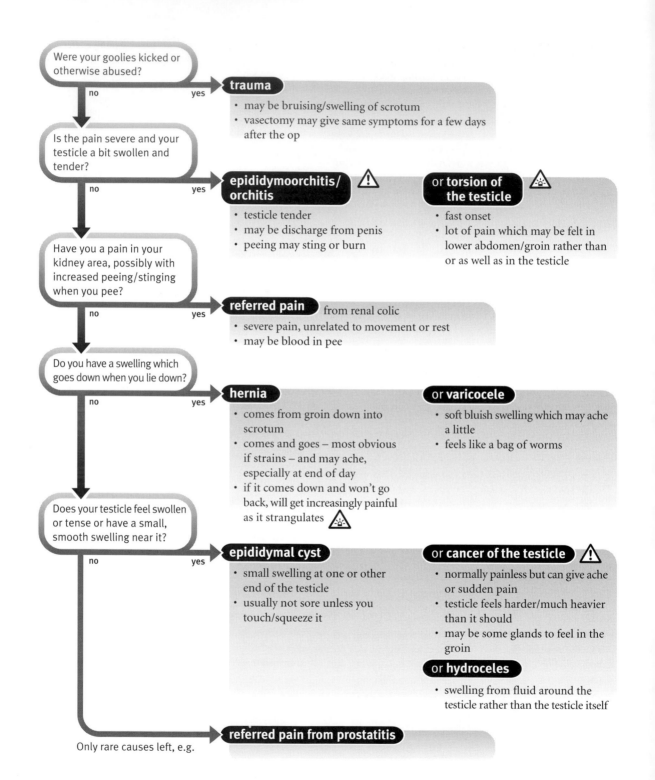

Were your goolies kicked or otherwise abused?

no · yes

trauma
- may be bruising/swelling of scrotum
- vasectomy may give same symptoms for a few days after the op

Is the pain severe and your testicle a bit swollen and tender?

no · yes

epididymoorchitis/ orchitis ⚠
- testicle tender
- may be discharge from penis
- peeing may sting or burn

or torsion of the testicle ⚠
- fast onset
- lot of pain which may be felt in lower abdomen/groin rather than or as well as in the testicle

Have you a pain in your kidney area, possibly with increased peeing/stinging when you pee?

no · yes

referred pain from renal colic
- severe pain, unrelated to movement or rest
- may be blood in pee

Do you have a swelling which goes down when you lie down?

no · yes

hernia
- comes from groin down into scrotum
- comes and goes – most obvious if strains – and may ache, especially at end of day
- if it comes down and won't go back, will get increasingly painful as it strangulates ⚠

or varicocele
- soft bluish swelling which may ache a little
- feels like a bag of worms

Does your testicle feel swollen or tense or have a small, smooth swelling near it?

no · yes

epididymal cyst
- small swelling at one or other end of the testicle
- usually not sore unless you touch/squeeze it

or cancer of the testicle ⚠
- normally painless but can give ache or sudden pain
- testicle feels harder/much heavier than it should
- may be some glands to feel in the groin

or hydroceles
- swelling from fluid around the testicle rather than the testicle itself

referred pain from prostatitis

Only rare causes left, e.g.

Epididymoorchitis The epididymis is a coiled tube, attached to the testicle, which collects sperm. If the epididymis and testicle get infected – usually by a sexually transmitted germ passing up the penis – the result is pain and swelling. This is epididymoorchitis.

Treatment This is explained in the 'Swelling in the scrotum' section (p. 133).

Orchitis This means inflammation of the testicle. It can affect one or both testicles, and the usual cause is a virus. The most well known is mumps, but this is rare nowadays because children are routinely immunized against this infection. Lots of other viruses, such as influenza, can inflame the testicles for a few days.

Treatment Check with your GP to make sure it's not epididymoorchitis, which needs antibiotics, or some other problem which he might need to treat. There's usually no particular medication needed for orchitis: just rest in bed (elevating the foot of the bed may ease the ache) and take painkillers while you're waiting for the problem to settle down. The good news is that this type of infection is highly unlikely to make you infertile.

Trauma We all know that an injury to the testicles is damn painful – anyone who's ever stepped on to a football field has probably experienced the agony of a ball in the balls. Very occasionally, a really nasty injury can damage the testicles or cause the scrotum (the ball-bag) to fill up with blood. The bruising which may follow a vasectomy is another form of trauma which can prove very uncomfortable.

Treatment The agony is usually over within a few minutes. If you've suffered a severe knock and the scrotum swells, then go to hospital for treatment. For discomfort after a vasectomy, use painkillers and ice-packs.

Torsion This is explained in the 'Swelling in the scrotum' section (p. 133). It's worth knowing that the pain starts before the swelling.

Treatment This is commoner in adolescents than adults. It can be difficult to tell apart from epididymoorchitis, but if in doubt, don't hang about – go straight to casualty. If it is a torsion, you've got about four hours before the testicle is 'dead'.

Referred pain This means pain coming from one place which is felt in another. Prostatitis (a germ in the prostate gland) and kidney stones can both cause pains 'referred' to the testicles.

Treatment Prostatitis is covered in the 'Blood in the sperm' section, and information about kidney stones is in the 'Renal colic' part of the 'Abdominal pain' sections (p. 13, p. 15).

Epididymal cyst, hydrocele, varicocele, hernia

These are all explained, and their treatments discussed, in the 'Swelling in the scrotum' section. They are likely to come to your attention more because of swelling rather than pain, but they can all cause a mild ache. Very rarely, a hernia can become 'strangulated' – in other words, throttled by the muscular weakness it's bulging through. If this happens, it will become very tender and you'll also get severe belly ache and vomiting – an urgent hospital job.

Cancer of the testicle Testicle cancer shows itself as a swelling in eight out of ten cases. It can cause pain, though – either a sudden, severe pain, or a nagging ache. Although it's the commonest type of growth in young men, it's still pretty rare. Further details about testicle cancer, and its treatment, are given in the 'Swelling in the scrotum' section (p. 133).

Palpitations

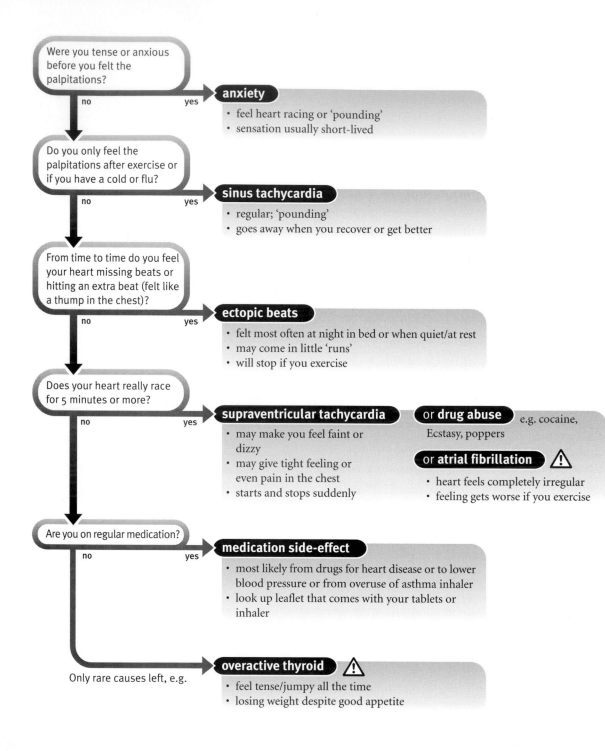

Were you tense or anxious before you felt the palpitations?

no   yes

anxiety
- feel heart racing or 'pounding'
- sensation usually short-lived

Do you only feel the palpitations after exercise or if you have a cold or flu?

no   yes

sinus tachycardia
- regular; 'pounding'
- goes away when you recover or get better

From time to time do you feel your heart missing beats or hitting an extra beat (felt like a thump in the chest)?

no   yes

ectopic beats
- felt most often at night in bed or when quiet/at rest
- may come in little 'runs'
- will stop if you exercise

Does your heart really race for 5 minutes or more?

no   yes

supraventricular tachycardia
- may make you feel faint or dizzy
- may give tight feeling or even pain in the chest
- starts and stops suddenly

or drug abuse e.g. cocaine, Ecstasy, poppers

or atrial fibrillation ⚠
- heart feels completely irregular
- feeling gets worse if you exercise

Are you on regular medication?

no   yes

medication side-effect
- most likely from drugs for heart disease or to lower blood pressure or from overuse of asthma inhaler
- look up leaflet that comes with your tablets or inhaler

Only rare causes left, e.g.

overactive thyroid ⚠
- feel tense/jumpy all the time
- losing weight despite good appetite

Palpitations

Anxiety People suffering from anxiety become more aware of their heartbeat and sometimes think their heart is racing or pounding even when it is beating perfectly normally. If you feel very tense, it's quite normal for the heart to beat faster than usual – most people notice this when they're in a situation which is making them nervous, such as making a speech. These sensations are often described as 'palpitations'.

Treatment It's important to realize that these sensations are harmless – otherwise, you might worry that there is something wrong with your heart, which will raise the anxiety levels even higher, causing more palpitations. If you're feeling tense most of the time, try to get to the root of the problem by sorting out the stressful areas of your life. Increasing your physical exercise, using relaxation techniques, and cutting down your caffeine intake (e.g. tea, coffee, and cola) may help. If the problem is causing you real difficulties and only happens in certain, predictable situations – such as when you have to give a presentation at work – it's worth seeing your GP. He might be able to advise about other relaxation techniques, or send you to see someone to help manage your anxiety. Or, if you're desperate, he might prescribe you something which will ease the palpitations and which you'll probably only have to take occasionally – whenever you're in the situation which brings on the palpitations.

Sinus tachycardia This is a heart which is beating appropriately fast. The normal rate is between 60 and 100 beats per minute. In sinus tachycardia, the rate is usually between 100 and 140 beats per minute. It happens, for example, after exercise or during a fever. The body needs more oxygen, so the heart pumps the blood around faster – hence the raised rate.

Treatment This is a normal response of the heart and so, in itself, does not require any treatment at all.

Ectopic beats The heart normally beats regularly, but it's quite normal for it to miss beats or throw in a few 'extra' beats occasionally. These odd irregular beats are not a sign of heart disease and are more noticeable, and sometimes more frequent, when you are stressed – they are the cause of the well-known 'butterflies in the stomach' sensation.

Treatment Usually, no specific treatment is needed – especially once you realize they're totally harmless. If they bother you, try the relaxation techniques outlined above.

It's also worth cutting down on caffeine, alcohol, and smoking, all of which may aggravate the problem.

Supraventricular tachycardia The heart contains its own natural pacemaker which keeps it beating at the usual rates. Occasionally, a temporary 'short circuit' occurs, resulting in the heart beating much faster than normal. As for most of the other causes of palpitations, it's not usually caused by any disease of the heart.

Treatment Most attacks stops within half an hour or so. If it lasts longer or makes you feel very unwell, then get someone to take you to hospital for treatment to slow the rate back to normal. Some people who get repeated attacks discover tricks which can stop an attack – these include sticking your fingers down your throat to make yourself gag, or quickly swallowing something very cold (such as a large lump of ice cream). There are tablets which can be taken to prevent attacks, so if you get repeated problems, see your GP, who will arrange any necessary tests and may start you on treatment.

Drug abuse Certain illicit drugs, such as cocaine, Ecstasy, poppers (amyl nitrite), and amphetamines, can make the heart race.

Treatment Although unpleasant, your racing pulse itself shouldn't cause you any problems – unless you already have heart trouble, which, in the under-45s, is unlikely. Obviously, the only way to cure these types of palpitation is to avoid the offending drug.

Medication side-effect A side-effect of some prescribed treatments is a speeding up of the heart rate. The most likely culprit is an asthma inhaler (such as salbutamol or terbutaline) – especially if it is used more often than recommended. Some blood pressure tablets can also cause palpitations.

Treatment If you feel that a prescribed medication you are taking might be causing palpitations, discuss the situation with your GP.

Overactive thyroid This is explained, and its treatment outlined, in the 'Excess sweating' section (p. 55).

Atrial fibrillation This involves the heart beating rapidly and irregularly. It is very rare in the under 45s, in whom excess alcohol is the likeliest cause.

Treatment This requires medication from your GP – and a reduction in alcohol intake if that is the cause.

Penis problems

NB This section contains a variety of problems which can affect your penis. For ulcers on the penis, discharge, and problems getting an erection, see the 'Penis sores and/or discharge' and 'Impotence' sections.

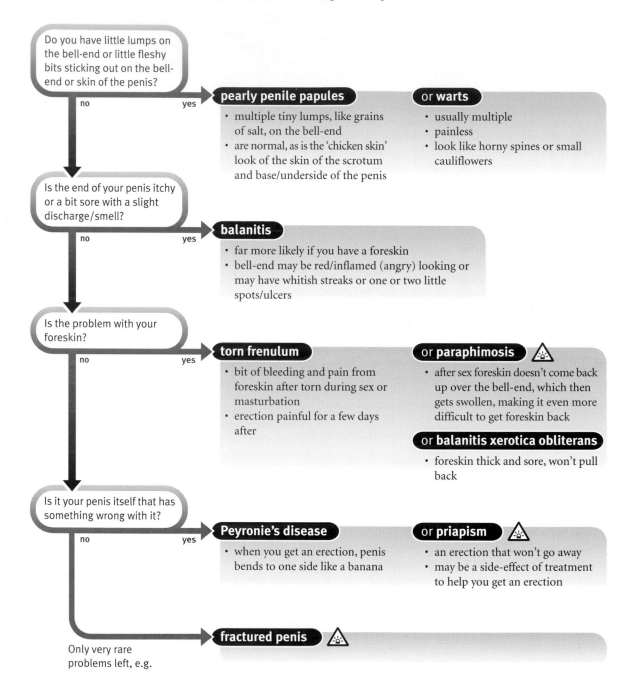

Do you have little lumps on the bell-end or little fleshy bits sticking out on the bell-end or skin of the penis?
no / yes

pearly penile papules
- multiple tiny lumps, like grains of salt, on the bell-end
- are normal, as is the 'chicken skin' look of the skin of the scrotum and base/underside of the penis

or warts
- usually multiple
- painless
- look like horny spines or small cauliflowers

Is the end of your penis itchy or a bit sore with a slight discharge/smell?
no / yes

balanitis
- far more likely if you have a foreskin
- bell-end may be red/inflamed (angry) looking or may have whitish streaks or one or two little spots/ulcers

Is the problem with your foreskin?
no / yes

torn frenulum
- bit of bleeding and pain from foreskin after torn during sex or masturbation
- erection painful for a few days after

or paraphimosis
- after sex foreskin doesn't come back up over the bell-end, which then gets swollen, making it even more difficult to get foreskin back

or balanitis xerotica obliterans
- foreskin thick and sore, won't pull back

Is it your penis itself that has something wrong with it?
no / yes

Peyronie's disease
- when you get an erection, penis bends to one side like a banana

or priapism
- an erection that won't go away
- may be a side-effect of treatment to help you get an erection

fractured penis

Only very rare problems left, e.g.

Pearly penile papules These are tiny lumps, each about the size of a grain of salt, on the bell-end ('glans') of your penis. There may be loads of them – but they're totally normal. They've probably been there for ages, but you might just have noticed them for the first time: maybe your partner has pointed them out, or you've had a one night stand and got anxious that you might have picked up an infection.

Treatment As they're normal – lots of blokes have them – they don't need any treatment. If you want to check that's what they are, ask your GP to take a quick peek.

Balanitis See the 'Penis sores and/or discharge' section (p. 107).

Warts Warts are caused by viruses – those which appear on your privates are usually passed on through sex.

Treatment Go to the 'special clinic' at your local hospital (it may be known by various other names, such as 'department of genitourinary medicine', 'sexually transmitted disease clinic', and the 'clap clinic'). Most hospitals have these clinics – just ring up and find out how soon they can see you. Get your partner checked too and wear a condom until they've been cured so you don't pass them on.

Torn frenulum The frenulum is the ridge of skin which joins the underside of the bell-end to the foreskin in men who've not been circumcised. This bit of skin can be quite tight, especially when you have an erection. Sometimes, during sex, it can get slightly torn, causing bleeding and pain. It heals up with a small scar which may make it tighter and can tear again.

Treatment If it's happened just once or twice, avoid sex for a couple of weeks to give it a chance to heal up. When you do try again, use a lubricant (like KY jelly) and a condom for a while – this helps prevent a further tear. If it keeps happening, though, see your GP – he'll probably refer you to a surgeon. You may end up with a small operation to lengthen the frenulum, or a circumcision (removal of the foreskin).

Peyronie's disease This is caused by a thickening of one side of the penis which makes it bend when it's erect.

Treatment Ignore a minor bend if you can. But if it's very painful or the bend makes sex impossible, see your GP – surgery can help.

Paraphimosis If men who haven't been circumcised don't roll their foreskin back after sex, they risk paraphimosis – the foreskin strangles the bell-end, which swells up and becomes very painful, making it impossible to get the foreskin back in place.

Treatment Go to casualty. They'll try to get the swelling down with ice-packs so they can roll your foreskin back. If that doesn't work, it's likely to mean a circumcision.

Balanitis xerotica obliterans In this condition, the foreskin thickens and gets sore, and it becomes impossible to pull it back. No one knows why it happens.

Treatment You'll need a circumcision, so see your GP, who'll arrange it for you.

Priapism This is an erection that won't go away. It's nowhere near as much fun as it sounds, as it's very painful and can damage the penis. It can be caused by blood problems or by medication used to treat impotence, but often just starts as a normal erection during sex which simply doesn't end up going limp when you've finished.

Treatment Forget the embarrassment and get to casualty quickly.

Fractured penis Yes, it can happen – it's basically a snap of the hard tissue of the erect penis, usually caused by over-gymnastic sex. But relax – it's very rare.

Treatment As for priapism (see above).

Penis sores and/or discharge

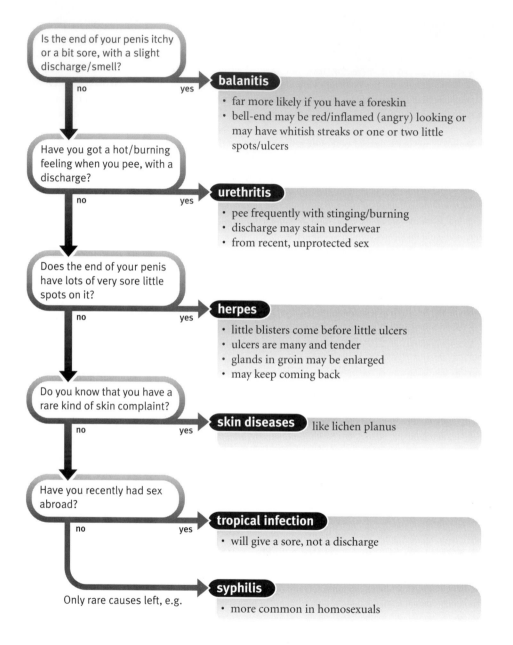

Is the end of your penis itchy or a bit sore, with a slight discharge/smell?

no / yes

balanitis
- far more likely if you have a foreskin
- bell-end may be red/inflamed (angry) looking or may have whitish streaks or one or two little spots/ulcers

Have you got a hot/burning feeling when you pee, with a discharge?

no / yes

urethritis
- pee frequently with stinging/burning
- discharge may stain underwear
- from recent, unprotected sex

Does the end of your penis have lots of very sore little spots on it?

no / yes

herpes
- little blisters come before little ulcers
- ulcers are many and tender
- glands in groin may be enlarged
- may keep coming back

Do you know that you have a rare kind of skin complaint?

no / yes

skin diseases like lichen planus

Have you recently had sex abroad?

no / yes

tropical infection
- will give a sore, not a discharge

Only rare causes left, e.g.

syphilis
- more common in homosexuals

Balanitis This means an inflamed bell-end (or 'glans'). It may just be itchy, or sore, or it may actually break out in sores. If you've not been circumcised, you might notice some discharge from under the foreskin. It's usually caused by thrush (a fungal infection), but can also be caused by a chemical, such as a bubble bath, irritating your penis.

Treatment Thrush can usually be cured by washing the sore area in plain water for a day or two. If this doesn't work, use some anti-thrush cream from the chemist, and if you've still not cured it, see your GP. Take a urine sample with you, because, very occasionally, severe thrush can be the first sign of diabetes – your GP can check this out with your sample of pee.

Urethritis The urethra is the tube in your penis which you pass urine through. Germs passed on during sex infect this tube, making it inflamed so that it stings when you have a pee. It can also leak some discharge. The germ is likely to be either Chlamydia, (causing 'non-specific urethritis', or 'NSU') or the gonorrhoea bug (causing 'the clap').

Treatment Go to the 'special clinic' at your local hospital (it may be known by various other names, such as 'department of genitourinary medicine', 'sexually transmitted disease clinic', and the 'clap clinic'). Most hospitals have these clinics – just ring up and find out how soon they can see you. It's worth getting your partner to go with you to get checked out too. You'll have a swab test taken from your urethra (a very thin cotton bud gently placed into the hole you pee out of) to work out which germ you have so that you can be given the right antibiotic. You'll probably also have further tests to see if you have any other sexually transmitted infections.

Herpes This is an infection caused by a virus. There are two sorts: the type which affects the genitals (passed on by having sex with an infected partner) and the type which causes cold sores. Sores on the penis are usually caused by the genital sort, but oral sex can lead to ulcers on the penis if your partner has a cold sore. The body does not totally get rid of the herpes virus, even if you've been given treatment. Because of this, it can come back – you've about a fifty-fifty chance of future attacks, although these won't be as bad as the first one, and they tend to get less frequent as time goes on.

Treatment Get to a 'special clinic' asap. They will give you treatment – usually tablets – and will check you out for any other sexually transmitted germs. If there's going to be a delay before you can be seen, discuss the situation with your GP – he may be able to start you off on treatment while you're waiting for your appointment. If you get attacks in the future, your GP or the doctors at the clinic will give you a cream to use. Very frequent attacks can sometimes be helped by taking tablets regularly for a while. It's worth wearing condoms once you know you've had herpes, otherwise you risk spreading the infection to your partner. You need to do this even if you're not having an attack, because the virus can be on your penis without you realizing it.

Skin diseases Some rare skin problems can cause ulcers on the penis. There may be spots or ulcers somewhere else on your body or it may just be your penis that's affected.

Treatment See your GP. He'll either sort the problem out himself, or if he's puzzled but thinks it could be a skin disease, he'll refer you to a skin specialist.

Tropical infections There are a number of diseases which can be picked up by having sex with a partner from a tropical country and which cause sores on the penis.

Treatment A 'special clinic' job.

Syphilis This is an infection with a special type of germ which is passed on through sex. It's rare these days and is most commonly seen in homosexuals.

Treatment Go to the 'special clinic' (see above). You'll be treated and followed up there, and checked out for any other sexually transmitted germs.

Pins and needles and numbness

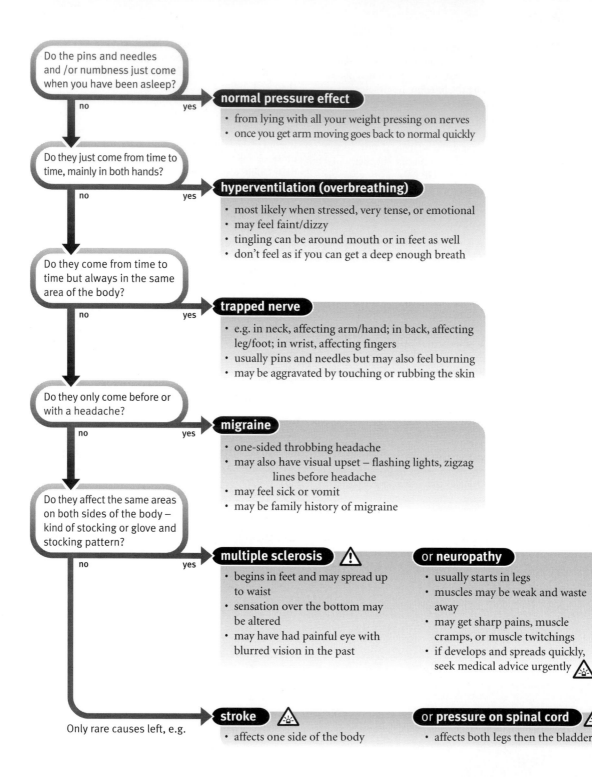

Do the pins and needles and /or numbness just come when you have been asleep?

no → yes →

normal pressure effect
- from lying with all your weight pressing on nerves
- once you get arm moving goes back to normal quickly

Do they just come from time to time, mainly in both hands?

no → yes →

hyperventilation (overbreathing)
- most likely when stressed, very tense, or emotional
- may feel faint/dizzy
- tingling can be around mouth or in feet as well
- don't feel as if you can get a deep enough breath

Do they come from time to time but always in the same area of the body?

no → yes →

trapped nerve
- e.g. in neck, affecting arm/hand; in back, affecting leg/foot; in wrist, affecting fingers
- usually pins and needles but may also feel burning
- may be aggravated by touching or rubbing the skin

Do they only come before or with a headache?

no → yes →

migraine
- one-sided throbbing headache
- may also have visual upset – flashing lights, zigzag lines before headache
- may feel sick or vomit
- may be family history of migraine

Do they affect the same areas on both sides of the body – kind of stocking or glove and stocking pattern?

no → yes →

multiple sclerosis ⚠
- begins in feet and may spread up to waist
- sensation over the bottom may be altered
- may have had painful eye with blurred vision in the past

or neuropathy
- usually starts in legs
- muscles may be weak and waste away
- may get sharp pains, muscle cramps, or muscle twitchings
- if develops and spreads quickly, seek medical advice urgently ⚠

Only rare causes left, e.g.

stroke ⚠
- affects one side of the body

or pressure on spinal cord ⚠
- affects both legs then the bladder

Key:
Favourites
Reasonable bets
Longer shots

Pins and needles and numbness

109

Normal pressure effect Most people have experienced waking in the night or first thing in the morning with a numb, 'dead', or tingly hand or arm, which comes back to normal after a minute or two. This is caused by the weight of your body temporarily trapping a nerve or affecting the circulation.

Treatment This is normal, harmless, and needs no treatment.

Hyperventilation This means breathing too fast and too deep and is usually part of a panic attack (see the 'Shortness of breath' section). You end up getting too much oxygen into your system, which affects your nerves, causing pins and needles.

Treatment The way to cure an attack is simply to breathe in and out of a brown paper bag. This way, you breathe back in your own air, which doesn't have so much oxygen in it as fresh air, so you don't overdose on oxygen. Also try to breathe slowly and not too deeply. It's very important that people around you understand that these attacks are harmless – if they panic, it'll make you worse. Getting panic attacks is usually brought on by stress – see the 'Shortness of breath' section (p. 123) for further advice on how to handle the problem.

Trapped nerve The nerves which supply feeling to your skin start from the spinal cord and then travel through various channels and tunnels in muscles and bones to reach their final destination. They can get pressed on (or 'trapped') at any point in their journey. The obvious example is when you hurt your 'funny bone' – a nerve passes through your elbow where you tend to knock it, so it's momentarily trapped, causing pins and needles in your hand. This goes away after a few seconds, but some nerves can be trapped for days or even weeks. Examples include nerves in the neck (causing problems in the arm and hand), nerves in the wrist (resulting in pins and needles in the palm and fingers), and a large nerve in the back (trapped when you slip a disc – 'sciatica' – causing numbness in your leg or foot).

Treatment A trapped nerve will usually sort itself out within a week or so. If it's painful or showing no signs of going, an anti-inflammatory drug like ibuprofen (available from the chemist) sometimes helps. But if it goes on for weeks without showing signs of improvement, gets worse, or causes weakness as well as numbness, see your GP – this will need checking out further and, if it is a trapped nerve, may need the help of a specialist to free it. For further information on sciatica, see 'Back pain' (p. 23).

Migraine This is explained in the 'Headache' section (p. 63). Before the blood vessels to the brain widen, causing the migraine, they sometimes narrow. This starves the brain of oxygen for a short while, with the result that you might feel numbness somewhere on one side of your body just before, or with, the headache.

Treatment See the 'Migraine' section of 'Headache' (p. 63).

Multiple sclerosis This is caused by the insulation around your nerves (which is just like the insulation around electrical wiring) dying off. Lots of different nerves can be affected, though not all at the same time, causing a variety of symptoms – including pins and needles or numbness – which usually come and go. What actually causes multiple sclerosis in the first place is still unknown.

Treatment If you think you have multiple sclerosis, you need to see your GP – but you're much more likely to have one of the other causes described above. If your GP is concerned, he'll refer you to a neurologist (a nerve specialist).

Neuropathy Lots of different medical problems can damage the nerves supplying the sensation to your skin, causing numbness or pins and needles. These include diabetes, excess alcohol, vitamin deficiencies, and some medications. Rarely, it may develop suddenly, perhaps a week or two after an infection (like a cold or tummy bug) and spread up your arms and legs and over the body. This is called Guillain–Barré syndrome.

Treatment See your GP. If he thinks you have a neuropathy, he'll run some blood tests to check it out, and will treat you according to what these tests show. If you think you might be developing Guillain–Barré syndrome, seek medical help urgently – this problem needs hospital treatment.

Other medical problems Some rare problems can cause pins and needles and numbness. These include strokes (which affect one half of the body, usually without a headache, for more than 24 hours) and problems in your spinal cord (which might make your legs go 'dead').

Treatment It's very unlikely that you'll have any of these problems. If you're concerned, see your GP.

Problems sleeping

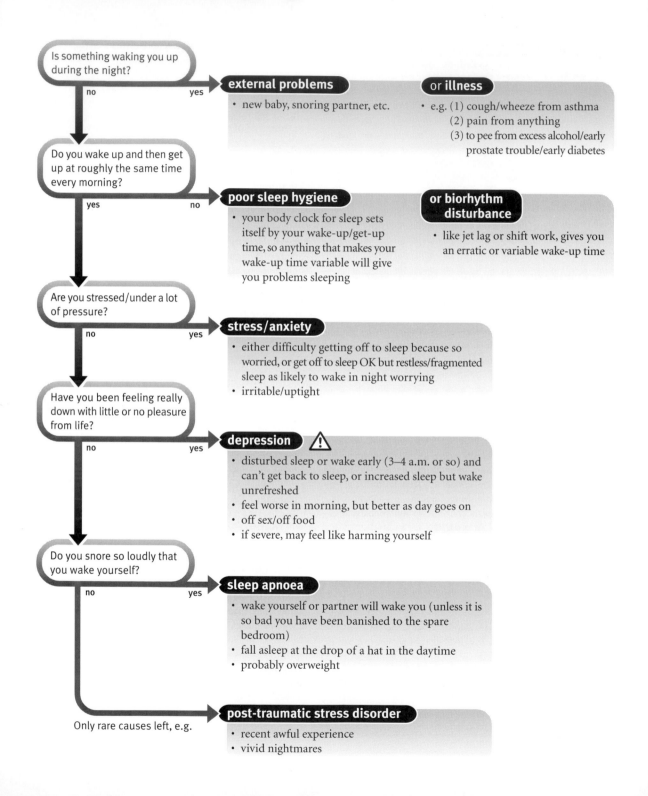

Is something waking you up during the night?

no → (down)
yes →

external problems
- new baby, snoring partner, etc.

or illness
- e.g. (1) cough/wheeze from asthma
  (2) pain from anything
  (3) to pee from excess alcohol/early prostate trouble/early diabetes

Do you wake up and then get up at roughly the same time every morning?

yes → (down)
no →

poor sleep hygiene
- your body clock for sleep sets itself by your wake-up/get-up time, so anything that makes your wake-up time variable will give you problems sleeping

or biorhythm disturbance
- like jet lag or shift work, gives you an erratic or variable wake-up time

Are you stressed/under a lot of pressure?

no → (down)
yes →

stress/anxiety
- either difficulty getting off to sleep because so worried, or get off to sleep OK but restless/fragmented sleep as likely to wake in night worrying
- irritable/uptight

Have you been feeling really down with little or no pleasure from life?

no → (down)
yes →

depression ⚠
- disturbed sleep or wake early (3–4 a.m. or so) and can't get back to sleep, or increased sleep but wake unrefreshed
- feel worse in morning, but better as day goes on
- off sex/off food
- if severe, may feel like harming yourself

Do you snore so loudly that you wake yourself?

no → (down)
yes →

sleep apnoea
- wake yourself or partner will wake you (unless it is so bad you have been banished to the spare bedroom)
- fall asleep at the drop of a hat in the daytime
- probably overweight

Only rare causes left, e.g.

post-traumatic stress disorder
- recent awful experience
- vivid nightmares

External problems Outside factors can stop you sleeping properly. These include being too cold or hot, the room not being dark enough, a snoring partner, or disturbances from your kids.

Treatment Getting your bedroom and bed as comfortable as possible will obviously help. Do this before you try to sleep rather than in the middle of the night. Wax ear plugs can help blot out the noise of a snoring partner. If your kids keep playing up at night, and so keeping you awake, check out one of the many books on taming your children, or discuss the problem with your health visitor (based at your GP's surgery).

Poor sleep hygiene Bad habits can mess up your sleep. These include too much caffeine (e.g. coffee, tea, and cola), regular alcohol, having an erratic routine, too much partying, illicit drugs, watching TV in bed, 'lying in' in the mornings, and taking naps during the day.

Treatment Sort out your lifestyle as best you can. A regular time for going to bed and waking, and avoiding dozing off during the day, are important. Exercising more will help. Don't try to zonk yourself out with booze, either – if used regularly, alcohol tends to disturb rather than help sleep. And in bed, don't toss and turn, watching the clock – if you really can't get to sleep, get up and do something for half an hour, then try again.

Stress and anxiety Feeling tense will make it hard for you to switch off, so you'll have trouble getting to sleep. You might also suffer from nightmares, which will aggravate the problem. The usual causes are worries about work, relationships, or money.

Treatment You'll find plenty of advice to help stress and anxiety in the 'Feeling tense' section (p. 59) and the 'Anxiety' part of the 'Palpitations' section (p. 103). Increasing your exercise helps cut stress levels – sex, in particular is an excellent way of relaxing which will help you sleep properly. Just tell your partner the doctor insisted. You might want to talk to your GP about the problem, but don't automatically expect sleeping pills. These are rarely prescribed these days because they don't help that much and can be addictive if used for more than a few weeks. Sometimes they're useful just for a few days to break a cycle of bad sleep.

Depression Depression can disturb your sleep by making you wake earlier in the morning than you'd planned. For details, see the 'Feeling down' section (p. 57).

Biorhythm disturbances Your body clock is usually set to follow the normal day/night pattern. It's not surprising, then, that messing it about – for example, through jet lag or shift work – will cause you problems sleeping.

Treatment If you're facing jet lag, make sure you don't drink too much booze on the plane, and sleep by your destination's time rather than by your body clock. Shift workers should set a regular sleep pattern, try to avoid being disturbed, and avoid the temptation to get up early to get things done during daylight hours. Sleeping tablets for a couple of days can occasionally be helpful in sorting out a biorhythm disturbance – discuss the situation with your GP.

Illness Various illnesses can disturb your sleep. These include any problem causing pain, asthma (if coughing or wheezing wake you), or waterworks problems.

Treatment The answer in this situation is to deal with the illness rather than the sleep problem – so speak to your GP.

Snoring/sleep apnoea Some blokes snore badly enough to disturb their own sleep, though this is more a problem in older men. A condition called 'sleep apnoea' causes earth-shattering snoring and can actually make you stop breathing for a short period in the night. You might regularly wake up coughing and spluttering and feel very dopey during the day. Your partner might tell you that your breathing seems to pack up in the night, or she might just leave you in disgust.

Treatment First, persuade your partner to try ear plugs. Next, slim down if you're overweight, and avoid alcohol late at night. If you're still in trouble, see your GP. There may be treatment to help, especially if you have sleep apnoea.

Post-traumatic stress disorder It's normal to have dreams or nightmares after an upsetting event. But if you've had some really awful experience, suffer vivid nightmares which disturb your sleep for more than a month and suffer other symptoms, you might have 'post-traumatic stress disorder' – a severe psychological reaction to an unpleasant event.

Treatment If the problem isn't getting better on its own, speak to your GP. He may treat you with antidepressants or refer you to a counsellor or psychiatrist.

Problems swallowing

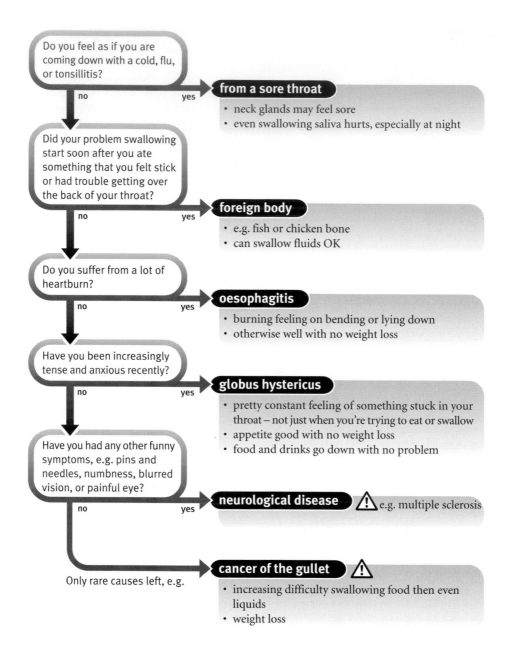

Do you feel as if you are coming down with a cold, flu, or tonsillitis?

no → (down)
yes → **from a sore throat**
- neck glands may feel sore
- even swallowing saliva hurts, especially at night

Did your problem swallowing start soon after you ate something that you felt stick or had trouble getting over the back of your throat?

no → (down)
yes → **foreign body**
- e.g. fish or chicken bone
- can swallow fluids OK

Do you suffer from a lot of heartburn?

no → (down)
yes → **oesophagitis**
- burning feeling on bending or lying down
- otherwise well with no weight loss

Have you been increasingly tense and anxious recently?

no → (down)
yes → **globus hystericus**
- pretty constant feeling of something stuck in your throat – not just when you're trying to eat or swallow
- appetite good with no weight loss
- food and drinks go down with no problem

Have you had any other funny symptoms, e.g. pins and needles, numbness, blurred vision, or painful eye?

no → (down)
yes → **neurological disease** ⚠ e.g. multiple sclerosis

Only rare causes left, e.g. → **cancer of the gullet** ⚠
- increasing difficulty swallowing food then even liquids
- weight loss

Remember: ⚠ means see your GP sharpish; ⚠ means an urgent hospital job

Problems swallowing

Sore throat of any cause If your throat is sore, then obviously it's going to be painful to swallow. For full details of the possible causes and treatment, see the 'Sore throat' section (p. 127).

Foreign body A bone or jagged-edged food (such as a bolted-down bag of chips) can scratch the throat, causing pain on swallowing. More rarely, a piece of bone can get stuck in the throat or gullet, causing discomfort and difficulty swallowing.

Treatment A scratch will heal with no treatment in a few days. If you think a piece of bone has got stuck, try eating some bread and drinking plenty of water, which may succeed in shifting it. If it persists, your best bet is to go to casualty to get it sorted out.

Oesophagitis The stomach contains acid to help digest your food. A valve at the top of the stomach prevents this acid from rising up ('refluxing') into the gullet. Sometimes, this valve does not work properly, with the result that acid coats and inflames your gullet ('oesophagitis'). You may feel this as an unpleasant burning feeling in the centre of your chest, especially on bending over or lying down (this is known as heartburn). Sometimes you can even taste the acid in your mouth. The inflamed area of the gullet may swell, causing pain on swallowing and, sometimes, a feeling that food sticks for a few seconds before it passes into the stomach.

Treatment Quick and easy cures are available from the chemist. These include antacid tablets and liquids to coat the gullet and neutralize the acid, and more powerful acid suppressants. But it's worth looking at your lifestyle too, otherwise the problem will tend to come back again. Try cutting down on cigarettes, alcohol (especially binges), and spicy foods, and avoid acidic tablets like aspirin and ibuprofen. Shed some pounds if you're overweight, eat sensibly and regularly, and try to avoid having anything to eat or drink within a couple of hours of going to bed – this tends to open up the valve, letting acid reflux into your gullet while you sleep. If you do tend to wake at night with heartburn, you may be able to cure the problem simply by raising the head of your bed by a few inches (a couple of bricks under the legs of your bed at the head end will do the trick) so that you sleep on a slight slope with your head higher than your feet. Don't just prop yourself up with pillows – this can actually make it worse. If all else fails, see your GP who will be able to prescribe powerful acid suppressants.

Globus hystericus When you swallow, your food goes down a muscular funnel – the 'pharynx' – which channels it into the gullet. If you're feeling tense, the muscles of the pharynx can contract. This causes a sensation of something stuck in the throat, often described as feeling like an apple core ('globus hystericus'). To get rid of this sensation, you'll tend to keep swallowing – unfortunately, this will make you focus on the symptom and may also make you worry that there is something seriously wrong. This, in turn, aggravates the tension and makes the symptom worse.

Treatment Half the battle is simply realizing that the symptom is caused by stress rather than anything sinister. This stops the vicious circle of tension causing the symptom causing more tension. Sorting out whatever in your life is getting you uptight is obviously important; making efforts to relax and taking some physical exercise will also help, see the 'Feeling tense' section (p. 59).

Neurological disease This means a disease of the nervous system (which controls and coordinates the body's sensation and movements). Diseases of this sort can affect the body in many ways, including how the muscles of the gullet coordinate and whether or not the valve at the entrance to the stomach opens properly. There are many different types and, fortunately, they're all very rare.

Treatment If your GP shares your concern, he'll refer you for tests.

Cancer Gullet cancer is very rare in the under 50s. Cancers of the lymph glands, which can cause trouble swallowing by pressing on the gullet, are more common, but highly unlikely to reveal themselves just with this particular symptom.

Treatment Discuss your symptoms with your GP, who will arrange any necessary tests or specialist appointments.

Problems with ejaculation

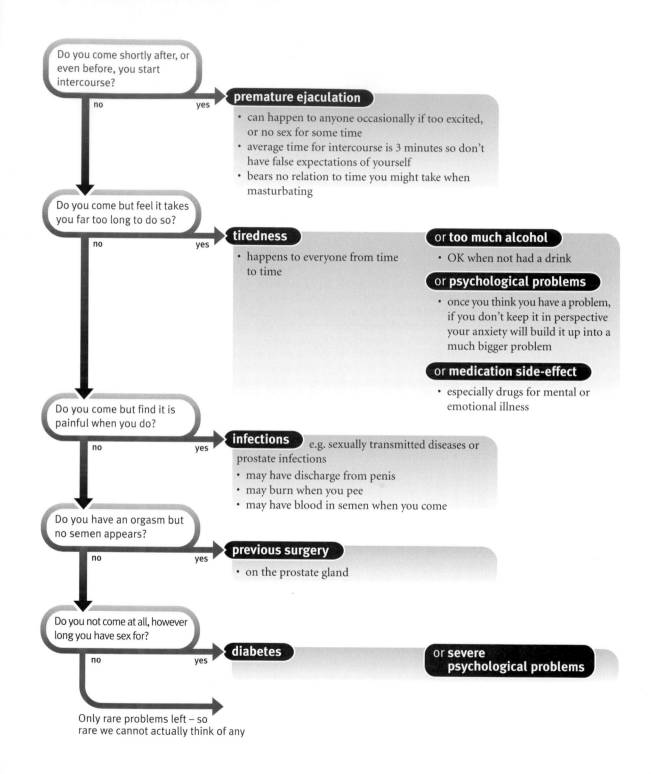

Do you come shortly after, or even before, you start intercourse?

no | yes

premature ejaculation
- can happen to anyone occasionally if too excited, or no sex for some time
- average time for intercourse is 3 minutes so don't have false expectations of yourself
- bears no relation to time you might take when masturbating

Do you come but feel it takes you far too long to do so?

no | yes

tiredness
- happens to everyone from time to time

or too much alcohol
- OK when not had a drink

or psychological problems
- once you think you have a problem, if you don't keep it in perspective your anxiety will build it up into a much bigger problem

or medication side-effect
- especially drugs for mental or emotional illness

Do you come but find it is painful when you do?

no | yes

infections e.g. sexually transmitted diseases or prostate infections
- may have discharge from penis
- may burn when you pee
- may have blood in semen when you come

Do you have an orgasm but no semen appears?

no | yes

previous surgery
- on the prostate gland

Do you not come at all, however long you have sex for?

no | yes

diabetes

or severe psychological problems

Only rare problems left – so rare we cannot actually think of any

Problems with ejaculation

Premature ejaculation This simply means coming too soon. How you define 'too soon' depends on the situation. Having your orgasm before you even enter your partner is obviously 'premature'. But you might still decide there is a problem if you have trouble satisfying your partner because she takes much longer to reach a climax than you do – so this, too, is a form of premature ejaculation. It boils down to the fact that men can come within two minutes of being sexually aroused, whereas for women it takes at least four times as long. If this mismatch isn't sorted out, and you keep ejaculating prematurely, sex can become a worry, which tends to aggravate the situation (this is known as 'performance anxiety').

Treatment The problem is often simply lack of experience. Most men come too soon when they first start having sex. If this is the situation you're in, try not to worry – anxiety will make it worse and it's likely to improve as you refine your sexual techniques. Just keep practising. If premature ejaculation keeps happening and it's starting to affect your relationship, the first thing to do is talk it over with your partner. Getting it out in the open can help defuse some of the tension and anxiety it causes. It's best to see it as a shared problem – avoiding being overexcited by your partner, while learning what really turns her on, will help you both achieve closer, more satisfying orgasms. One practical way around the problem is to use foreplay to bring her very close to coming, and only then actually penetrate her with your penis. Mild premature ejaculation may be helped by wearing a condom (or two) or using a local anaesthetic cream (available from the chemist) to numb the penis slightly.

If you're getting nowhere with the problem, then try the 'squeeze' technique. A firm squeeze of your penis with finger and thumb just below the bell-end (the 'glans') just when you think you're about to come can stop you climaxing. This can be repeated as often as necessary, while you continue to stimulate your partner, so your climax can be delayed until you're both 'ready'. In time, your body helps to control itself, without the squeeze. You can also practise this yourself, during masturbation. There are many books and videos available giving more details about these, and similar, techniques. If all else fails, your GP may be able to offer further advice or may refer you and your partner to a sex therapist.

Tiredness Being knackered can stop or delay your ejaculation.

Treatment Don't worry – this is quite normal. Explain to your partner that you're just tired and don't dwell on it, or you may develop 'performance anxiety', which in itself can affect ejaculation, creating a vicious cycle.

Too much alcohol If it doesn't stop you getting a hard-on, it may make it difficult for you to ejaculate because it can numb the penis.

Treatment Go easy on the booze before sex.

Psychological problems Any anxiety can delay or stop your ejaculation. For example, you might think the neighbours can hear you or you could be worried about getting your partner pregnant.

Treatment Get to the root of whatever's worrying you and avoid the vicious cycle of performance anxiety (discussed above).

Medication side-effect Some prescribed drugs, such as antidepressants, can make it difficult for you to ejaculate.

Treatment Check the patient information leaflet supplied with the treatment. If ejaculation problems are mentioned, speak to your GP to see if you still need the medication, or if you could be switched to something else.

Infections The urethra – the tube in the penis you pass urine and sperm through – can get infected (usually with sexually transmitted germs – see 'Penis sores and discharge'). The same can happen to the prostate gland (see 'Prostatitis' in the 'Blood in sperm' section). Both can make your orgasm painful.

Treatment See the 'Penis sores and discharge' and 'Blood in sperm' sections.

Previous surgery Operations on the prostate gland can make the sperm spurt up into your bladder (it passes out in your urine later) rather than out into your partner. This is called 'retrograde ejaculation'.

Treatment This type of surgery is almost never performed in men under 45, so it's highly unlikely that this is your problem. Retrograde ejaculation caused by surgery is harmless, but cannot be treated.

Diabetes This is explained in the 'Impotence' section (p. 69). Very occasionally, diabetes can damage the nerves which coordinate ejaculation, so you may take a long time to come or you may not come at all.

Treatment The treatment of diabetes is outlined in the 'Impotence' section.

Rash

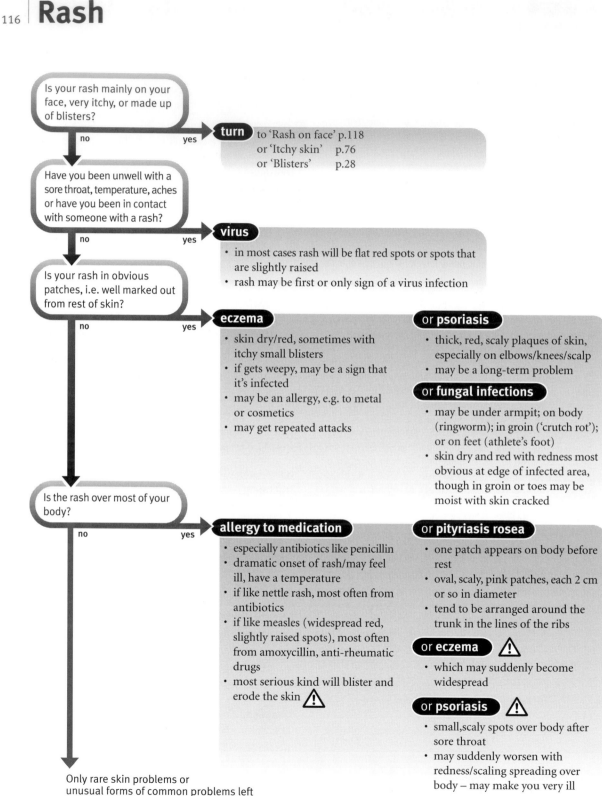

Is your rash mainly on your face, very itchy, or made up of blisters?

no → yes

turn to 'Rash on face' p.118
or 'Itchy skin' p.76
or 'Blisters' p.28

Have you been unwell with a sore throat, temperature, aches or have you been in contact with someone with a rash?

no → yes

virus
- in most cases rash will be flat red spots or spots that are slightly raised
- rash may be first or only sign of a virus infection

Is your rash in obvious patches, i.e. well marked out from rest of skin?

no → yes

eczema
- skin dry/red, sometimes with itchy small blisters
- if gets weepy, may be a sign that it's infected
- may be an allergy, e.g. to metal or cosmetics
- may get repeated attacks

or psoriasis
- thick, red, scaly plaques of skin, especially on elbows/knees/scalp
- may be a long-term problem

or fungal infections
- may be under armpit; on body (ringworm); in groin ('crutch rot'); or on feet (athlete's foot)
- skin dry and red with redness most obvious at edge of infected area, though in groin or toes may be moist with skin cracked

Is the rash over most of your body?

no → yes

allergy to medication
- especially antibiotics like penicillin
- dramatic onset of rash/may feel ill, have a temperature
- if like nettle rash, most often from antibiotics
- if like measles (widespread red, slightly raised spots), most often from amoxycillin, anti-rheumatic drugs
- most serious kind will blister and erode the skin ⚠

or pityriasis rosea
- one patch appears on body before rest
- oval, scaly, pink patches, each 2 cm or so in diameter
- tend to be arranged around the trunk in the lines of the ribs

or eczema ⚠
- which may suddenly become widespread

or psoriasis ⚠
- small, scaly spots over body after sore throat
- may suddenly worsen with redness/scaling spreading over body – may make you very ill

Only rare skin problems or unusual forms of common problems left

Virus A rash is just one of the many symptoms (like fever and sore throat) that a virus produces as it works its way through your system.

Treatment There's no magic cure for a virus. Try paracetamol if you feel hot and achy, and calamine lotion if the rash is itchy. It usually disappears after a few days. It's best to steer clear of women who are (or might be) pregnant until you're better – you can never be sure what type of virus you have, and some might harm the baby. For more information about chickenpox and shingles – caused by one particular type of virus – see the 'Blisters' section.

Eczema/dermatitis This is explained, and its treatment outlined, in the 'Itchy skin' section (p. 77).

Psoriasis The layers of your skin usually replace themselves every month. If you have psoriasis, your skin for some reason goes into overdrive, causing patches of thickening and scaling. It sometimes runs in families.

Treatment Like eczema, patches may come and go or it may affect your skin constantly. Moisturizers and creams or lotions containing coal tar can help (available from the chemist). See your GP if you're getting nowhere, as there are lots of other effective treatments – and if necessary, he can refer you to a dermatologist (a skin specialist).

Fungal infections Athlete's foot is an infection caused by a fungus. Similar infections can occur on other areas of the skin, especially where it's moist, such as the armpit or groin (known as 'crutch rot').

Treatment Keep the areas clean and dry and get an antifungal cream from the chemist.

Pityriasis rosea This is quite common, especially in adolescents and young adults in autumn and winter. It is possibly due to a virus, although it's not infectious.

Treatment No treatment is needed – it goes away on its own, though it may take a few weeks. If it's a bit irritating, try a moisturizer from the chemist.

Allergy to medication Any medication – prescribed or over the counter – can cause an allergic rash, but the most likely culprits are antibiotics, aspirin, or anti-inflammatory drugs like ibuprofen. The type of rash varies, but it can be 'urticaria' (see the 'Itchy skin' section, p. 77). You might not make the connection between the rash and the medication – you may have taken the treatment before without any problem, or the rash may take three weeks from the first dose to appear.

Treatment Stop the treatment which has caused the rash and don't take it again. Also, let your doctor know what has happened (just leave him a message) so the allergy goes on your medical records. The rash usually goes within a few days. If you have urticaria, take the advice given in the 'Urticaria' part of the 'Itchy skin' section.

Unusual skin problems There are a number of rare skin problems. Also, the rashes of even the more common skin diseases are sometimes not typical.

Treatment Check out your rash with your GP. If he's stuck for an answer and it's a nuisance to you, he'll probably refer you to a dermatologist.

Rash on the face

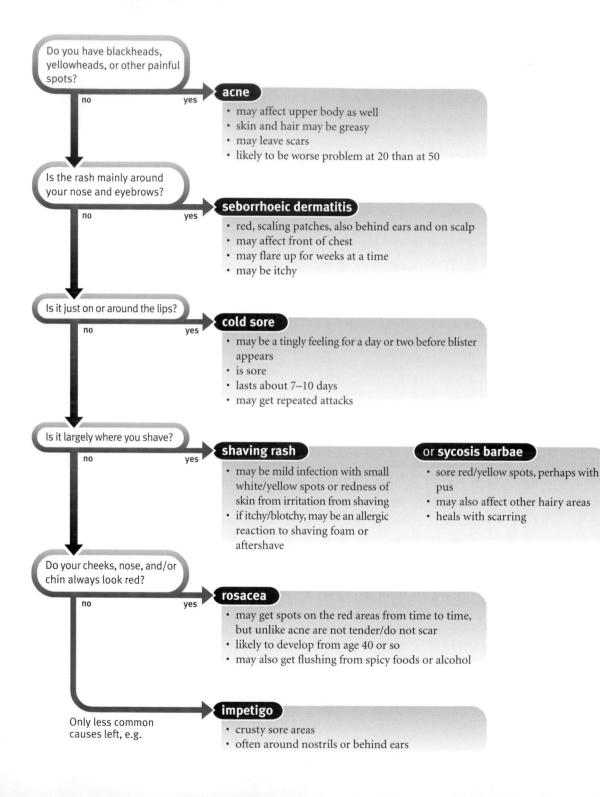

Do you have blackheads, yellowheads, or other painful spots?

no → yes →

acne
- may affect upper body as well
- skin and hair may be greasy
- may leave scars
- likely to be worse problem at 20 than at 50

Is the rash mainly around your nose and eyebrows?

no → yes →

seborrhoeic dermatitis
- red, scaling patches, also behind ears and on scalp
- may affect front of chest
- may flare up for weeks at a time
- may be itchy

Is it just on or around the lips?

no → yes →

cold sore
- may be a tingly feeling for a day or two before blister appears
- is sore
- lasts about 7–10 days
- may get repeated attacks

Is it largely where you shave?

no → yes →

shaving rash
- may be mild infection with small white/yellow spots or redness of skin from irritation from shaving
- if itchy/blotchy, may be an allergic reaction to shaving foam or aftershave

or sycosis barbae
- sore red/yellow spots, perhaps with pus
- may also affect other hairy areas
- heals with scarring

Do your cheeks, nose, and/or chin always look red?

no → yes →

rosacea
- may get spots on the red areas from time to time, but unlike acne are not tender/do not scar
- likely to develop from age 40 or so
- may also get flushing from spicy foods or alcohol

Only less common causes left, e.g.

impetigo
- crusty sore areas
- often around nostrils or behind ears

Rash on the face

Acne This is very common and is, to some extent, a normal part of adolescence. It may not disappear until your mid 20s and sometimes happens in older age groups. It's caused by the glands which produce the normal grease on your skin getting blocked. This results in 'blackheads', and infection of the stagnant grease leads to the inflamed pus-spots characteristic of acne. When very severe, it can cause large cysts and scarring.

Treatment Mild acne needs no treatment at all if it doesn't bother you. Getting out in the sunshine helps (though avoid overdoing it or getting sunburnt), but messing around with your diet won't make any difference. It's important to keep your skin clean to remove excess grease and reduce the germs which aggravate the problem. You'll find some effective treatments available over the counter: for example, benzoyl peroxide (cream, gel, or lotion) can help a lot. It may cause stinging or redness at first – use the lowest strength, sparingly, at first, then increase the strength and how often you use it as your skin gets used to it. If this doesn't work, or your acne is severe – especially if you're getting cysts or scarring – see your GP. He can prescribe a number of effective treatments (such as antibiotics) and, if they don't work, or your acne is really bad, he may refer you to a dermatologist (a skin specialist) for more powerful treatment.

Seborrhoeic dermatitis The cause is thought to be an infection with a fungus. The rash can affect other areas, such as your scalp, chest, groin, and armpits.

Treatment You should be able to sort this out using an anti-fungal cream (such as clotrimazole, available from the chemist), which is perfectly safe to use on the face. The rash can come back – just use the cream as and when you need to. If the scalp is affected, it's important to clear that up too by using an anti-fungal shampoo regularly – sorting out the scalp often helps the rash on the face (see the 'Itchy scalp' section).

Cold sore This is caused by a virus (the herpes simplex virus). Once you've had an attack, the virus never fully leaves you – it lies dormant in a nerve and can reactivate at certain times, resulting in repeated attacks, nearly always in the same area (usually the lip). There may be no particular trigger for attacks but stress, being run down, and sunlight may bring them on.

Treatment There is no 'cure' to get rid of the virus once and for all. Some people find that using a cream from the chemist – aciclovir – at the first sign of an attack can help a bit.

Shaving rash Redness of the beard area after shaving can be caused by an allergy to shaving cream or aftershave. Or you may just have very sensitive skin which is irritated by the use of a razor or electric shaver.

Treatment Any cool, soothing moisturizer from the chemist may help. Otherwise, it's a case of experimentation: try different shaving foams or different ways of shaving (if you wet shave, try an electric razor, and vice versa). If all else fails, you can either put up with it or grow a beard.

Rosacea The cause for this combination of pus spots, redness, and flushing is unknown. It usually starts in your 40s.

Treatment Alcohol, hot drinks, and spicy foods can aggravate the flushing, so you may want to avoid, or cut down, these. Otherwise, there's not much you can do in the way of self-treatment – and don't use hydrocortisone from the chemist, as this makes it worse. If the problems is a real nuisance, see your GP, as he can prescribe effective treatment such as antibiotic creams or tablets.

Impetigo This is an infection of the skin by a particular type of germ. It may get into the skin through a cut or graze, or it may infect some other skin problem, such as eczema or a cold sore.

Treatment A mild attack may be sorted out with an antiseptic cream. Otherwise, you'll need to see your GP for antibiotics in the form of a cream or capsules.

Sycosis barbae This is an infection of the beard area.

Treatment See your GP for some antibiotics. If you keep getting attacks, wash your face and neck regularly with an antiseptic soap and keep your shaving gear clean.

Red eye

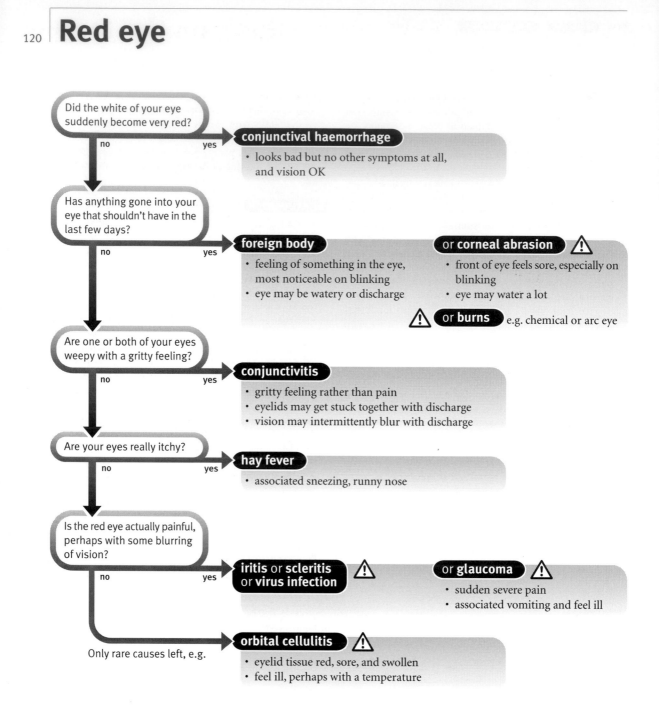

Did the white of your eye suddenly become very red?

no / **yes** → **conjunctival haemorrhage**
- looks bad but no other symptoms at all, and vision OK

Has anything gone into your eye that shouldn't have in the last few days?

no / **yes** → **foreign body**
- feeling of something in the eye, most noticeable on blinking
- eye may be watery or discharge

or corneal abrasion ⚠
- front of eye feels sore, especially on blinking
- eye may water a lot

⚠ **or burns** e.g. chemical or arc eye

Are one or both of your eyes weepy with a gritty feeling?

no / **yes** → **conjunctivitis**
- gritty feeling rather than pain
- eyelids may get stuck together with discharge
- vision may intermittently blur with discharge

Are your eyes really itchy?

no / **yes** → **hay fever**
- associated sneezing, runny nose

Is the red eye actually painful, perhaps with some blurring of vision?

no / **yes** → **iritis or scleritis or virus infection** ⚠

or glaucoma ⚠
- sudden severe pain
- associated vomiting and feel ill

Only rare causes left, e.g. → **orbital cellulitis** ⚠
- eyelid tissue red, sore, and swollen
- feel ill, perhaps with a temperature

Remember: ⚠ means see your GP sharpish; ⚠ means an urgent hospital job

Conjunctivitis The eye has a delicate cling-film wrapper type covering: the conjunctiva. When this gets infected, usually from a cold, it becomes reddened and discharges mucky pus – this is conjunctivitis.

Treatment A mild, early case can be cured with gentle, regular bathing of the eye using cotton wool soaked in warm water. If it's not getting any better, or the eyes are really sticky and sore, see your GP for some antibiotic eye ointment.

Hay fever Allergy to pollen causes hay fever. The eyes alone may be affected, or they may just be part of the overall runny nosed, sneezing misery.

Treatment Simple measures include avoiding long walks when the pollen count is high (usually early morning and evening), wearing sunglasses to reduce glare, and keeping the car windows wound up (otherwise the car acts as a pollen trap). It's worth a trip to the chemist: various eye-drops, or antihistamine tablets, can help a lot.

Foreign body A bit of dirt or debris on the eye or under the lids will cause irritation.

Treatment If something has simply blown into the eye, get someone to gently remove it with the corner of a hanky. There are a couple of tricks you can use to sort out something caught under the upper lid. Try turning the lid inside out – you can do this by grasping the eyelashes in one hand, and using a cotton bud in the other to gently push on the upper surface of the lid, rolling the lid around the bud. Your accomplice should now be able to fish out the offending piece of dirt. If you're on your own, try pulling the upper lid down, by the lashes, over the lower lid, then releasing. As the upper lid returns to its normal position, the lower lid lashes may sift out the foreign body. Tiny pieces of metal from grinding can stick on the front of the eye or even enter the eye itself. Get it checked at casualty.

Corneal abrasion A scratch on the front of the eye. This is usually caused by a minor injury – like from a twig or a baby's fingernail – or a foreign body (see above).

Treatment See your GP. He will assess the damage and probably treat you with antibiotic ointment. If it doesn't heal quickly – usually within a day or two – you may need to see an opthalmologist (an eye specialist).

Conjunctival haemorrhage A leak of blood in the conjunctiva. It usually appears for no obvious reason, but may be caused by violent coughing or retching.

Treatment Despite its dramatic appearance, it needs no treatment at all – it's perfectly harmless and disappears within a few days.

Iritis Inflammation of the coloured part of the eye (the iris). It is sometimes connected to rare types of arthritis.

Treatment See your GP – he'll probably send you to an eye specialist urgently to get it checked out and for treatment with eye drops. The problem can recur: your specialist is likely to tell you what action to take should you get further problems.

Burns Chemicals splashed into the eye can result in burns. So too can arc welding – if goggles aren't used, it causes a flash burn.

Treatment If a chemical has splashed into your eye, wash it out with lots of water, then go to casualty for further treatment (try to take the name of the chemical with you). For arc eye, see your GP for treatment with drops – and wear goggles in future.

Virus: Herpes simplex or shingles Herpes simplex is the virus which causes cold sores. Rarely, it can infect the eye, causing ulcers and inflammation. Shingles is caused by a similar virus and can also affect the eye (see the 'Blisters' section for more details).

Treatment Another GP job and likely to need urgent specialist treatment if confirmed.

Scleritis Inflammation of the white of the eye. Like iritis, it can be linked to joint problems (such as rheumatoid arthritis).

Treatment Check with your GP – you're likely to need to see an eye specialist.

Orbital cellulitis An infection of the hole – the orbit – in which the eye sits, which usually then spreads to the eye itself.

Treatment Can get very nasty if not treated quickly with antibiotics. See your GP, who may send you to hospital.

Acute glaucoma A sudden increase in the pressure of the fluid in the eye. Very rare in the under 50s.

Treatment If your GP thinks you have got acute glaucoma, which is pretty unlikely, he'll send you straight to the eye specialist.

Shortness of breath

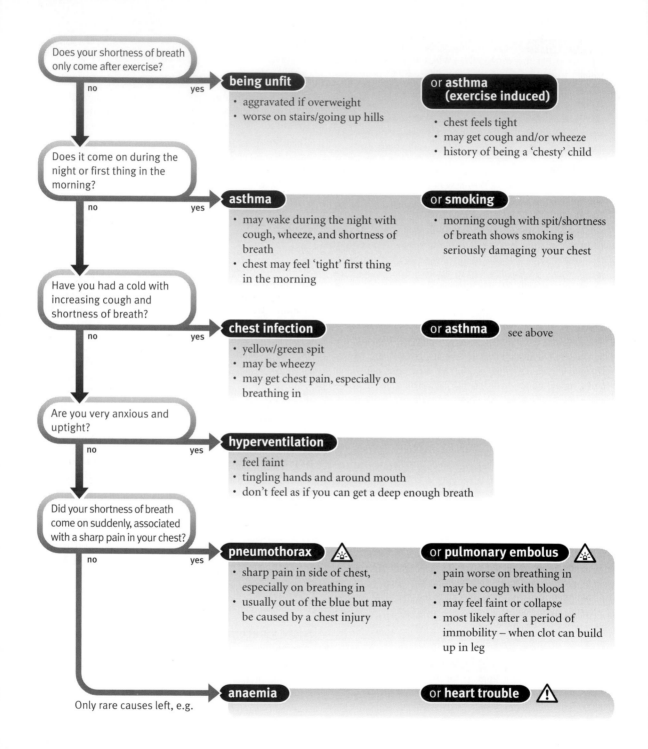

Does your shortness of breath only come after exercise?

no / yes

being unfit
- aggravated if overweight
- worse on stairs/going up hills

or asthma (exercise induced)
- chest feels tight
- may get cough and/or wheeze
- history of being a 'chesty' child

Does it come on during the night or first thing in the morning?

no / yes

asthma
- may wake during the night with cough, wheeze, and shortness of breath
- chest may feel 'tight' first thing in the morning

or smoking
- morning cough with spit/shortness of breath shows smoking is seriously damaging your chest

Have you had a cold with increasing cough and shortness of breath?

no / yes

chest infection
- yellow/green spit
- may be wheezy
- may get chest pain, especially on breathing in

or asthma see above

Are you very anxious and uptight?

no / yes

hyperventilation
- feel faint
- tingling hands and around mouth
- don't feel as if you can get a deep enough breath

Did your shortness of breath come on suddenly, associated with a sharp pain in your chest?

no / yes

pneumothorax ⚠
- sharp pain in side of chest, especially on breathing in
- usually out of the blue but may be caused by a chest injury

or pulmonary embolus ⚠
- pain worse on breathing in
- may be cough with blood
- may feel faint or collapse
- most likely after a period of immobility – when clot can build up in leg

anaemia

or heart trouble ⚠

Only rare causes left, e.g.

Shortness of breath

Being unfit and/or overweight If you've let yourself get out of shape, you're bound to feel more short of breath than usual after you've run up a few flights of stairs. You'll notice it even more if you're overweight, simply because you're effectively carrying excess baggage around all the time.

Treatment Get your bottom off the couch and down the gym. Break yourself back in gently, though – if you go hell for leather from the start you risk injuring yourself or making yourself ill. Gradually improve your level of fitness and aim for about three sessions of exercise of around half an hour each week (enough to make you sweat). This will help you shed excess pounds, too, as will a revamp of your diet.

Smoking Everyone knows that cigarette smoke can permanently damage the lungs and aggravate other lung conditions (such as asthma – see below). It also lowers the levels of oxygen in the blood, narrows the airways, and reduces the volume of your lungs.

Treatment Cut down, and preferably give up, the ciggies. Only do this when you feel really motivated because otherwise you'll fail which may make you believe you can never succeed. Get as much help as you can – read a leaflet or book on how to give up, persuade your partner to stop too, and get all fags and ashtrays out of the house. Make sure the Big Day is during a phase when you're not too stressed, and then just stop – don't mess around trying to wean yourself off them. Staying stopped is the really tricky bit. Avoid situations which prompt you to have a fag, and consider using nicotine replacement if you get really bad cravings (available from the chemist as a gum, patch, or nose spray). You're very likely to need nicotine treatment if you light up first thing in the morning or smoke more than 20 a day, and the chemist can explain how you should use it. And don't worry if you put on weight – you can sort that out once you're over the ciggies. Most blokes who manage to give up do so with simple advice and maybe nicotine replacement treatment. A few use other measures such as hypnotherapy, but you may be better off taking a long hard look at why you've failed to give up, and trying to put it right, than spending money on a miracle cure. If you don't *really* want to stop, then no treatment on earth is going to help you kick the habit.

Asthma This is explained, and the treatment discussed, in the 'Cough' section (p. 43).

Chest infection See the 'Cough' section (p. 43).

Hyperventilation If you don't think you're getting enough air into your lungs, you'll tend to breathe deeper or faster – this is hyperventilation. It is usually caused by anxiety, because tension tends to tighten up the muscles of the rib cage so that you feel your chest isn't expanding enough. A vicious cycle builds up because the feeling of breathlessness increases the anxiety, tensing up the muscles even more. A sudden, severe attack is known as a 'panic attack'.

Treatment Try to get to the root of the problem by sorting out the main stresses in your life. Relaxation therapy can help (whatever switches you off) and physical exercise will also burn off nervous energy. A panic attack can be helped by making sure that those around you know what's going on (otherwise they'll panic too, making you worse), trying to stay calm, and breathing in and out of a paper bag. If you seem to be getting nowhere, see your GP – he may be able to sort out anxiety management sessions for you. Very occasionally, you might need medication, especially if your hyperventilation is a part of depression (see 'Feeling down' section).

Pneumothorax This is a collapsed lung. Air suddenly escapes into the gap between the lung and the ribs, squashing the lung. It usually happens for no particular reason – blokes (especially tall, thin ones) are about five times as likely as women to suffer this, and it's also more common in asthmatics. It can also be caused by an injury, like a broken rib or a stab wound.

Treatment If you think you might have a pneumothorax, your best bet is to go straight to casualty.

Other medical conditions A whole heap of other problems can cause breathlessness. These include anaemia, heart valve problems, chronic bronchitis, angina, and a pulmonary embolus (a blood clot on the lung). Fortunately, none are likely to apply to you.

Treatment If the shortness of breath is sudden and severe, go straight to hospital. Otherwise, make an appointment with your GP.

Skin marks and lumps

Are patches of – not spots on – your skin a different colour from normal?
no / yes

vitiligo
- pale/white patches, most obvious if rest of your skin is coloured/tanned

or tinea versicolor
- most noticeable on front of chest/armpits
- shows as 'dirty' areas on pale skin/paler areas on dark or tanned skin

Do you have a lump under the skin rather than on it?
no / yes

sebaceous cyst
- may be anywhere except palms/soles
- usually only one, slow growing, softish to feel
- may give smelly, cheesy discharge

or ganglion
- hard, smooth, round swelling on back of hand or top of foot

or lipoma
- softish lump under the skin

Do your skin bumps look warty – raised and rough?
no / yes

warts
- look different depending on which part of the body they are on, e.g. on hands look like proper warts; on feet like small corns; on face or genitals like horny spines or small cauliflowers

or molluscum contagiosum
- most often on trunk or genital area
- pearl coloured, dome shaped with a central crater

or seborrhoeic warts
- develop as you get older
- not usually single, light brown – evenly coloured, seem as if they are stuck on to the skin surface

Do they/it look like a mole – brown or black?
no / yes

benign mole
- uniform colour, even surface
- unchanging or very slowly growing (over years)

or histiocytoma
- mostly on limbs
- often light brown, firm, and hard, seem deeply set in the skin

or melanoma ⚠
- irregular colour or black
- irregular surface
- grow over weeks or months
- surface may become eroded or crusted
- surrounding skin may become pigmented

Do they/it look red?
no / yes

Campbell de Morgan spots
- sign of approaching middle age!
- small, multiple, bright red, mainly on the trunk

or pyogenic granuloma
- red, shiny nodule which may appear suddenly
- bleeds easily so often that covered by dark scab

Other causes left include

skin tags
- small and may be single or multiple – tiny tags of skin

or xanthelasma/xanthoma
- yellow, fatty looking lumps around the eyes, elbows, or knees

or other types of skin cancer ⚠
- especially on face, back, hands, legs
- may be pigmented or crusty or form a 'horn' of hard skin
- may seem to heal then come back then heal again

⚠ **Any coloured skin mark which is changing colour or size or which bleeds easily, should be checked by a doctor.**

Benign moles Little clusters of the cells in the skin which produce pigment.

Treatment They can be left alone but need to be distinguished from 'melanoma' (see the flow chart).

Warts/molluscum contagiosum (NB For information about warts on the penis, see the 'Penis problems' section) Warts are caused by a virus and can occur anywhere, especially on the hands and feet (where they're known as verrucas). Molluscum contagiosum are similar, and are also caused by a virus. If they appear on your privates or lower belly, they may have been passed on sexually.

Treatment Warts eventually go on their own, although they can take years. If you want to get rid of them, use a lotion from the chemist to soften the skin, then rub with a pumice stone – but this may take weeks to work. If you're really desperate, see your GP, who might arrange to have them frozen off. Warts on your privates – and around the back passage, which can be passed on sexually in homosexuals – need special assessment and treatment (see the 'Penis problems' section). Molluscum contagiosum go on their own eventually. You can speed things up by pricking them with a sterile needle – or you can see your GP, who might freeze them off.

Skin tags Tiny extra flaps of skin. What causes them is unknown.

Treatment These can be left alone. If you want to get rid of them, see your GP.

Sebaceous cyst If one of the glands which produces the grease on your skin gets blocked, the grease can't escape and so forms a lump – a sebaceous cyst.

Treatment These are harmless and so don't need any treatment. A cyst can be removed if it's a nuisance – see your GP, who will sort it out (a very simple minor operation).

Campbell de Morgan spots Numerous small red spots which develop in your late 30s or early 40s.

Treatment None required as they're completely normal.

Vitiligo This makes the pigment-producing cells of your skin pack up. The cause is unknown, and it sometimes runs in families.

Treatment Unfortunately, most people with vitiligo are stuck with it. Many of the treatments tried don't achieve much, though you may want to discuss this with your GP. It's important to use sunblocks in the summer – the problem will look much worse if your 'normal' skin tans. Camouflage cosmetics can help a lot if you're desperate.

Ganglion A hard, fluid-filled lump which develops over a joint. The cause is unknown.

Treatment They're safe to leave alone. They can be cut out, but it's not a small operation and it might come back.

Lipoma A fatty lump under the skin, cause unknown.

Treatment It's safe to leave well alone.

Seborrhoeic keratosis A warty overgrowth of skin. They're much commoner in the elderly, but they can occur in young blokes.

Treatment Totally harmless; they can be frozen off if they're a nuisance.

Xanthelasma/xanthoma Collections of fat (xanthelasma occurs around the eyes and xanthoma on the elbows or knees). They are sometimes caused by a high cholesterol level in your blood.

Treatment None is needed, but it's worth getting your cholesterol level checked.

Pyogenic granuloma A small skin lump, probably caused by a very minor injury.

Treatment See your GP to get it checked and, if necessary, removed.

Histiocytoma A tiny skin lump – possibly the result of an old insect bite.

Treatment None needed.

Tinea versicolor An infection with a type of fungus.

Treatment Anti-fungal creams from the chemist will usually cure the problem, but you may need to use them for a few weeks. Selenium sulphide shampoo (available over the counter) can also help. Apply once a week for eight weeks, then wash it off after a few hours. Use it on your scalp, too, as the fungus may live in your hair and then reinfect your skin. This rash can cause patches of your skin to lighten – this can take months to improve, even after treatment.

Melanoma This is a skin cancer developing from the cells which produce pigment – it can sometimes start in a mole. In blokes, it usually happens in the 30–50 age range, and is most common on the back. The cause is thought to be exposure to sunlight (especially severe episodes of sunburn in childhood).

Treatment See your GP asap. If he thinks you might have a melanoma, he'll refer you to a dermatologist (a skin specialist).

Other skin cancers These are unusual in young blokes and, again, are probably linked to sun exposure.

Treatment See your GP, who will refer you to a dermatologist.

Sore throat

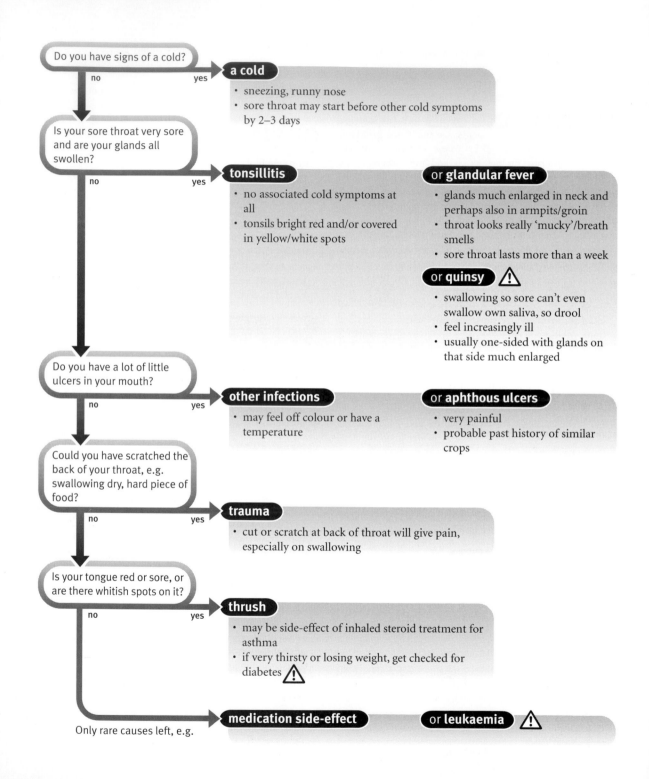

Do you have signs of a cold?

no / yes

a cold
- sneezing, runny nose
- sore throat may start before other cold symptoms by 2–3 days

Is your sore throat very sore and are your glands all swollen?

no / yes

tonsillitis
- no associated cold symptoms at all
- tonsils bright red and/or covered in yellow/white spots

or glandular fever
- glands much enlarged in neck and perhaps also in armpits/groin
- throat looks really 'mucky'/breath smells
- sore throat lasts more than a week

or quinsy ⚠
- swallowing so sore can't even swallow own saliva, so drool
- feel increasingly ill
- usually one-sided with glands on that side much enlarged

Do you have a lot of little ulcers in your mouth?

no / yes

other infections
- may feel off colour or have a temperature

or aphthous ulcers
- very painful
- probable past history of similar crops

Could you have scratched the back of your throat, e.g. swallowing dry, hard piece of food?

no / yes

trauma
- cut or scratch at back of throat will give pain, especially on swallowing

Is your tongue red or sore, or are there whitish spots on it?

no / yes

thrush
- may be side-effect of inhaled steroid treatment for asthma
- if very thirsty or losing weight, get checked for diabetes ⚠

Only rare causes left, e.g.

medication side-effect

or leukaemia ⚠

A cold Colds are infections caused by viruses which irritate the upper part of the airways – this includes the ears, nose, and throat.

Treatment There is no cure for a cold, so there's no point in seeing your GP. Antibiotics don't help at all. The symptoms settle on their own after a few days – your throat will be helped by soluble aspirin gargles or paracetamol, and plenty of fluids.

Tonsillitis The tonsils are two lumps of gristle which are part of the immune system and which sit in your throat, one on each side of the dangly bit (the 'uvula'). When infected by bacteria, they become swollen, painful, and either red like a strawberry or covered with pus.

Treatment Even the docs can't decide on this one. Some GPs will always give antibiotics, some don't prescribe them at all, but most make a judgment on each individual case. Research shows that, if antibiotics help, all they do is speed up recovery by a day or two. If the attack is mild and you feel reasonably well, try the self- help measures mentioned under 'A cold'. If your throat is very sore, you're feverish, and feeling terrible, then it's worth contacting your GP.

Glandular fever This is a type of virus, usually passed on by close contact. It causes symptoms very similar to tonsillitis. In some cases, the throat can become very sore, causing difficulty in swallowing, and you might continue to feel out of sorts for some weeks after the soreness has disappeared.

Treatment Some doctors will arrange a blood test to confirm that you have glandular fever. This isn't always necessary, though – your GP may make the diagnosis just by looking at your throat, and point out that it's simply a virus which lasts a bit longer than most. Or you may have such a mild attack that you don't bother to see your GP at all. Besides, there's no specific treatment for this problem other than the simple measures outlined above. So knowing you've got glandular fever doesn't help much, apart from providing an explanation as to why your throat might feel sore – or you feel lousy – for longer than usual. The rare case which makes it impossible to swallow and makes you feel dreadful does need medical attention, of course.

Trauma A swallowed bone or badly chewed food – especially chips or crisps – can scratch the back of the throat, causing an area of soreness.

Treatment Just take painkillers if necessary, drink plenty of fluids, and chew your food carefully so as not to aggravate it – it'll heal in a few days.

Qunisy This is an abscess around one tonsil – an unusual complication of tonsillitis.

Treatment See your GP. An early one may be cured by antibiotics. But if the abscess is fully developed, you'll need to go to hospital to have it lanced under anaesthetic.

Other infections There are a number of other germs – mainly viruses – which can cause a sore throat. Often, they produce lots of small, painful ulcers which can also appear on the lips, gums, and tongue.

Treatment All that's usually needed is the standard treatment of aspirin gargles or paracetamol and plenty of cool fluids. It's only worth seeing your GP if it's making you feel very ill or you're having trouble swallowing any fluids because of the pain.

Thrush This is a fungus infection. The most common problem it produces is infection of the vagina in women, which results in itching and discharge – but it can affect the throat too, in either sex.

Treatment Get some anti-fungal lozenges or medicine from your GP. This problem is unusual in the under 45s – the likeliest cause in this age group is a side-effect of asthma inhalers. Steroid inhalers tend to encourage the thrush fungus to grow in the throat. If you have asthma and you use this type of treatment, try to improve your inhaler technique (check the patient leaflet supplied with the inhaler) and gargle some water after each dose. Your GP may prescribe a 'spacer' – a gizmo which attaches to your inhaler and directs the spray into your lungs rather than the back of your throat. Rarely, in people not on asthma inhalers, thrush infection of the throat may be a sign of diabetes or an immune problem – your GP may check out these possibilities.

Aphthous ulcers These are explained in the 'Mouth ulcers' section (p. 87). As they can occur anywhere in the mouth, they are sometimes the cause of a sore patch in the throat.

Treatment There is no cure, but you can try various gels and pastes from the chemist which, if used early, can help clear up an attack – but it can be tricky applying it to the throat as it'll tend to make you gag.

Medical rarities There are some rare medical problems which can cause a persistent and severe sore throat – these include serious blood disorders and the side-effects of some treatments (such as some anti-thyroid or anti-epilepsy drugs).

Treatment If you think you fit into this category, which is highly unlikely, see your GP to get the problem checked out.

Stiff or painful neck

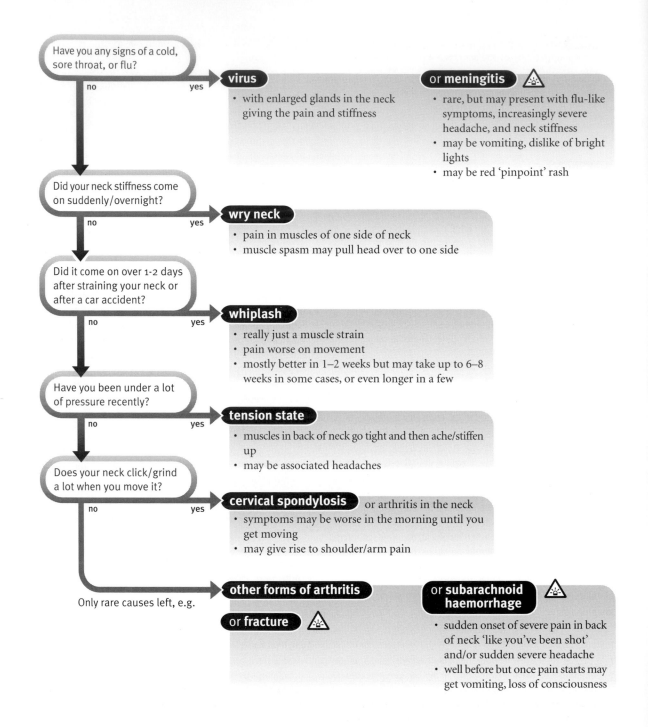

Have you any signs of a cold, sore throat, or flu?

no / yes

virus
- with enlarged glands in the neck giving the pain and stiffness

or meningitis
- rare, but may present with flu-like symptoms, increasingly severe headache, and neck stiffness
- may be vomiting, dislike of bright lights
- may be red 'pinpoint' rash

Did your neck stiffness come on suddenly/overnight?

no / yes

wry neck
- pain in muscles of one side of neck
- muscle spasm may pull head over to one side

Did it come on over 1-2 days after straining your neck or after a car accident?

no / yes

whiplash
- really just a muscle strain
- pain worse on movement
- mostly better in 1–2 weeks but may take up to 6–8 weeks in some cases, or even longer in a few

Have you been under a lot of pressure recently?

no / yes

tension state
- muscles in back of neck go tight and then ache/stiffen up
- may be associated headaches

Does your neck click/grind a lot when you move it?

no / yes

cervical spondylosis or arthritis in the neck
- symptoms may be worse in the morning until you get moving
- may give rise to shoulder/arm pain

Only rare causes left, e.g.

other forms of arthritis

or fracture

or subarachnoid haemorrhage
- sudden onset of severe pain in back of neck 'like you've been shot' and/or sudden severe headache
- well before but once pain starts may get vomiting, loss of consciousness

If you get a sudden severe pain in the back of your neck or increasing headache and neck stiffness, seek medical help immediately to exclude subarachnoid haemorrhage or meningitis.

Stiff or painful neck

Virus with enlarged glands in the neck When you have a virus causing a sore throat or flu, the glands in your neck may swell. This is a sign that your body's immune system is fighting off the germ. The enlarged glands can irritate the neck muscles, resulting in stiffness.

Treatment You're unlikely to need much more than some paracetamol or aspirin, plenty of fluids, and some sympathy.

Wry neck This is spasm of the neck muscles. It may be caused by a trapped nerve in the neck or by sleeping in an awkward position. The muscles cramp up, causing pain, stiffness, and sometimes pulling your head over to one side.

Treatment Try heat, massage, and painkillers from the chemist, and get the neck moving as quickly as possible. The problem usually sorts itself out within a couple of days. A rare type, called 'spasmodic torticollis', keeps coming back and occasionally needs specialized treatment – so see your GP if you get repeated attacks of wry neck.

Tension state If you are uptight, your muscles tend to tense up – particularly in the neck. This causes a constant dull ache and stiffness.

Treatment Massage, heat, and neck exercises usually work well; you can use over-the-counter painkillers if necessary too. Also, try to get to the root of the problem – either by sorting out whatever it is in your life that's getting you tense, or by winding down more. Getting fitter and trying relaxation exercises will help.

Whiplash This results from a sudden stretching of the neck muscles. They become inflamed, leading to pain and stiffness which often doesn't appear until a day or so after the injury. A typical cause is a car accident in which you are shunted in the rear: your head suddenly jerks back, then forwards, like the 'crack' of a whip.

Treatment The key thing is to get your neck moving as quickly as possible. As it may be very stiff and painful, you may need regular and strongish painkillers – ask your pharmacist for advice. As with most stiff necks, massage and heat will also help. Many people find wearing a soft collar effective, but be warned: research shows that, if the collar is worn for more than a couple of days, the stiffness takes longer to settle. So if you have been given a collar, get rid of it as soon as possible, grit your teeth, and exercise that neck. While most whiplash injuries get better quickly, a few take months, or even longer, to heal. X-rays don't help at all, and other treatments like physiotherapy usually make very little difference.

Cervical spondylosis The spine, including the neck, is made up of a column of small bones which interlock with each other via lots of very small joints. As you get older, these joints suffer wear and tear (osteoarthritis). In the neck, this is known as cervical spondylosis. It can result in a clicking, grinding neck with attacks of pain and stiffness.

Treatment All the treatments already mentioned will also help this problem. Again, neck exercise is important to relieve stiffness. Anti-inflammatory drugs such as ibuprofen (available from the chemist) can be very effective. Cervical spondylosis is sometimes worse in the morning, probably because you accidentally twist your neck into uncomfortable positions during the night. A butterfly pillow – a specially shaped headrest which can easily be made by tying some string tightly around the middle of a pillow so that it forms a 'bow tie' shape – can help by keeping your head still at night.

Other forms of arthritis Special types of arthritis such as rheumatoid arthritis and ankylosing spondylitis, which affect various joints and, sometimes, other parts of the body too, can cause trouble in the neck.

Treatment Your GP will probably try you on anti-inflammatory drugs, but you are also likely to be referred to a rheumatologist (a joint specialist) for further treatment.

Fracture A severe injury, such as diving into shallow water and bashing your head on the bottom of the pool, can break one of the small bones in the neck. Not surprisingly, this will cause severe pain and neck spasm.

Treatment You are unlikely to have to worry about self-treatment too much – chances are, you're already in hospital.

Meningitis This is an inflammation of the lining of the brain. One of its effects is to send the neck muscles into spasm, so it's difficult to flex your head – in other words, to get your chin on to your chest. It's serious, but rare, and if you're unfortunate enough to be suffering from meningitis, you're likely to be complaining of rather more than a stiff neck.

Treatment Straight to hospital without delay.

Subarachnoid haemorrhage This is explained in the 'Headache' section (p. 63). Like meningitis, it inflames the brain lining, causing a stiff neck.

Swelling in the groin

Have you felt lumps in both groins?

- no
- yes

Are they small (pea sized) and not at all tender to touch?

- no
- yes

normal glands

- do not change size with time

abnormal glands from infection

- if quick onset and sore throat may be glandular fever
- if at risk of having caught a sexually transmitted disease, may be from that

or abnormal glands from cancer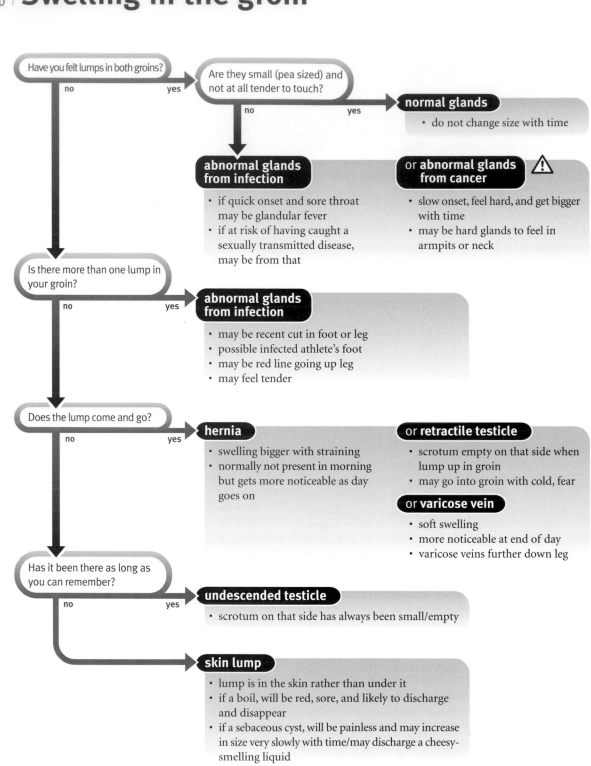

- slow onset, feel hard, and get bigger with time
- may be hard glands to feel in armpits or neck

Is there more than one lump in your groin?

- no
- yes

abnormal glands from infection

- may be recent cut in foot or leg
- possible infected athlete's foot
- may be red line going up leg
- may feel tender

Does the lump come and go?

- no
- yes

hernia

- swelling bigger with straining
- normally not present in morning but gets more noticeable as day goes on

or retractile testicle

- scrotum empty on that side when lump up in groin
- may go into groin with cold, fear

or varicose vein

- soft swelling
- more noticeable at end of day
- varicose veins further down leg

Has it been there as long as you can remember?

- no
- yes

undescended testicle

- scrotum on that side has always been small/empty

skin lump

- lump is in the skin rather than under it
- if a boil, will be red, sore, and likely to discharge and disappear
- if a sebaceous cyst, will be painless and may increase in size very slowly with time/may discharge a cheesy-smelling liquid

Normal glands Glands are found in various part of the body – particularly the neck, the armpits, and the groin. They are a part of your immune system, which helps fight off infections. If you're slim, it's quite normal to be able to feel these glands as pea-sized, non-tender lumps which stay roughly the same size most of the time.

Treatment Being able to feel these glands is entirely normal, so no treatment is needed.

Abnormal glands from infection Sometimes, the 'normal' glands in the groin described above can swell because a germ has got into your body. Causes include germs which enter the body near the groin (such as an infected cut on the leg or a sexually transmitted disease), or other bugs which make all the glands swell (like glandular fever – see the 'General infection' part of the 'Swollen glands' section, p. 139).

Treatment This obviously need careful checking by your GP, who will treat the infection which has made the glands swell.

Hernia This is a bulge of the gut through a muscle weakness. It's common in men and may be brought on, or made worse by, heavy lifting, being overweight, being constipated, and coughing a lot.

Treatment The only effective treatment for a hernia is an operation. This is usually a fairly small job, often performed as a 'day case' (in other words, you're in and out of hospital on the same day). It's worth getting done if the hernia aches or otherwise bothers you – in which case, see your GP, who'll arrange it for you. Rarely, a hernia can strangulate. This means that it gets throttled by the surrounding muscles, resulting in the swelling becoming very tender, hard, and 'irreducible' – it doesn't disappear with firm pressure or on lying down. A strangulated hernia will also block the bowel, causing belly ache, swelling of the abdomen, and vomiting. If you think your hernia is strangulating then get to the hospital asap.

Retractile testicle Muscles can pull the testicles up into the groin. As a result, at times, one or both testicles can be felt not in the wrinkled bag of skin they're usually found in (the scrotum), but in the groin. Once whatever has triggered the muscle contraction has gone – and it may be cold, fear, being touched, or even tight trousers – the testicles will go back down to their normal resting place.

Treatment This is quite normal and requires no treatment.

Skin lump (various types) The skin can develop a variety of different lumps, and any of these can be found in the groin. Especially common are sebaceous cysts (blocked glands which produce the grease on our skin), lipomas (small collections of fat), and boils or abscesses (infections causing a small swelling full of pus).

Treatment Most of these swellings are totally harmless and are best left alone. If they're caused by infection, they normally enlarge and become tender, in which case you will need either antibiotics or the swelling lanced – speak to your GP.

Varicose vein A varicose vein is a swollen, twisting vein, usually found in the leg. Severe varicose veins can start from the groin, producing a noticeable swelling – the rest of the vein may be more difficult to feel.

Treatment Varicose veins rarely cause any problems. If they ache or look terrible, they can either be treated with a tight stocking or with an operation – but they often tend to come back again after surgery. If you can't just put up with them, discuss the problem with your GP.

Abnormal glands from cancer Very rarely, serious diseases (such as lymph gland cancers) can make the glands in the groin slowly get larger, and may affect other glands as well.

Treatment A GP job. If he suspects a serious cause like cancer, he'll refer you urgently to a hospital specialist.

Undescended testicle Your testicles actually started life somewhere near your kidneys, in the lower part of your back. As you developed from fetus into fully grown baby, they descended down, through the abdomen, and into your scrotum. In a few men, they get stuck (undescended) or misplaced (ectopic) along the way and so never appear in the scrotum, but may be felt in the groin (do not confuse this with the much more common – and normal – retractile testicles).

Treatment It's highly unlikely that this is your problem – most undescended or ectopic testicles are spotted during babyhood or childhood. If you're concerned, see your GP, as it's important to sort it out if you really do have this problem. The treatment will involve an operation.

Swelling in the scrotum

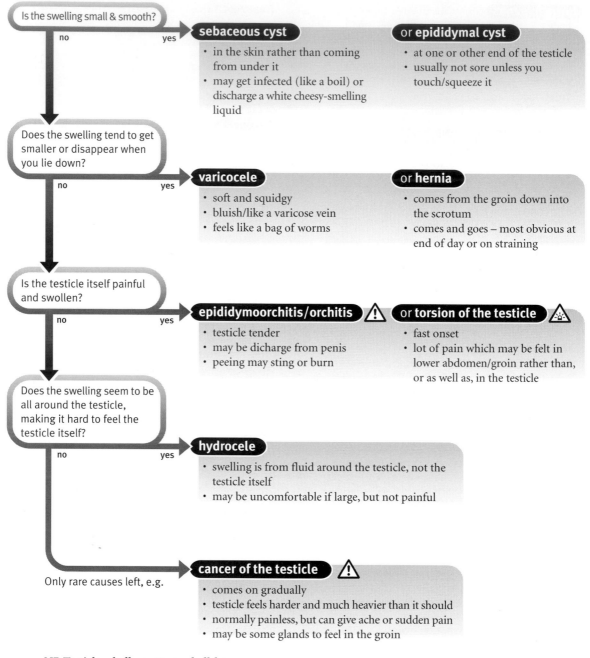

Is the swelling small & smooth? — no / yes

sebaceous cyst
- in the skin rather than coming from under it
- may get infected (like a boil) or discharge a white cheesy-smelling liquid

or epididymal cyst
- at one or other end of the testicle
- usually not sore unless you touch/squeeze it

Does the swelling tend to get smaller or disappear when you lie down? — no / yes

varicocele
- soft and squidgy
- bluish/like a varicose vein
- feels like a bag of worms

or hernia
- comes from the groin down into the scrotum
- comes and goes – most obvious at end of day or on straining

Is the testicle itself painful and swollen? — no / yes

epididymoorchitis/orchitis ⚠
- testicle tender
- may be discharge from penis
- peeing may sting or burn

or torsion of the testicle ⚠
- fast onset
- lot of pain which may be felt in lower abdomen/groin rather than, or as well as, in the testicle

Does the swelling seem to be all around the testicle, making it hard to feel the testicle itself? — no / yes

hydrocele
- swelling is from fluid around the testicle, not the testicle itself
- may be uncomfortable if large, but not painful

Only rare causes left, e.g.

cancer of the testicle ⚠
- comes on gradually
- testicle feels harder and much heavier than it should
- normally painless, but can give ache or sudden pain
- may be some glands to feel in the groin

NB Testicle = ball; scrotum = ball-bag

⚠ Although cancer of the testicle is a long shot, if you're in any doubt about a swelling in the scrotum, get it checked asap by your GP.

Sebaceous cyst The sebaceous glands produce the oil which keeps our skin healthy. If one gets blocked, a small lump – a sebaceous cyst – develops in the skin. The scrotum is a common site.

Treatment Forget it, it's harmless. If you don't like the look of it, or it keeps getting infected – when it will keep turning into a type of boil – then you could consider getting it cut out under local anaesthetic, but it might come back again.

Epididymal cyst Between the testicle, which makes sperm, and the spermatic cord, which carries it to the penis, is a coiled tube which acts as a sperm departure lounge – the epididymis. This can fill with fluid and swell, producing an epididymal cyst.

Treatment Much as above, but a slightly more complex operation if you opt for the knife – usually a 'day case' at your local hospital.

Varicocele A collection of varicose veins – swollen blood vessels – in the scrotum.

Treatment Probably best left alone. Some doctors believe that a varicocele can affect fertility (the warm blood in the veins increases the testicle's temperature, making the sperm sleepy – or so the theory goes), but the jury is still out on this one. If you suffer from infertility and have a varicocele then your doctor *might* think it's worth getting sorted – usually with a small operation.

Orchitis and epididymoorchitis Orchitis means an inflamed testicle. This is usually caused by a virus – typically mumps, though this is pretty rare nowadays. Epididymoorchitis – where the testicle and epididymis are infected – is more common. The most likely cause is a sexually transmitted germ travelling up the penis and into the epididymis.

Treatment See your GP as you are likely to need antibiotics. Ice-packs, painkillers, and lying in bed with the foot of the bed raised will help ease the pain. It's worth knowing that the swelling can take ages to go down, although the pain usually settles quickly. And relax: these infections do not make you infertile.

Hernia A bulge of gut through a muscular weakness. A big one can travel down into the scrotum, producing a lump.

Treatment Only one way to sort this out – an operation. So see your local doc, who will arrange it for you.

Hydrocele A collection of fluid around the testicle. This may happen for no particular reason, but it can be the result of some problem with the testicle itself.

Treatment The fluid needs to be drained off so the testicle can be checked properly. This is either a hospital or GP job – so the first stop is your local surgery. Very occasionally, a hydrocele keeps coming back. In this case, an operation can cure the problem.

Torsion If the spermatic cord twists, the blood supply to the testicle is cut off. This is bad news because, with no blood, the testicle will die in about four hours – so it lets you know all about it by causing sudden severe pain and swelling.

Treatment It can be difficult to distinguish from epididymoorchitis (see above) – even the doc may have trouble telling the two apart. If in doubt, don't 'wait and see' because, if it is torsion, time is of the essence – go straight to casualty.

Cancer of the testicle Cancer of the testicle is the commonest type of growth in men aged 20–40. But it's still pretty rare – each year, you only have around a 1 in 25 000 chance of developing it.

Treatment See your GP asap. He'll refer you urgently to a specialist. The good news is that testicular cancer has a fantastic cure rate, particularly if spotted early – so any lump in the scrotum you're not absolutely sure is harmless should be checked by your GP. This is one of the few occasions where it's very sensible to be ultra-cautious.

Swelling of the breast

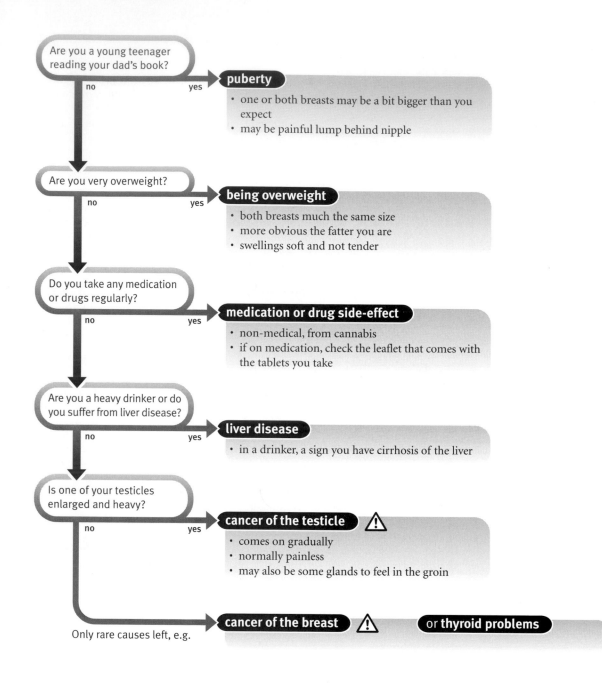

Are you a young teenager reading your dad's book?

no / yes

puberty
- one or both breasts may be a bit bigger than you expect
- may be painful lump behind nipple

Are you very overweight?

no / yes

being overweight
- both breasts much the same size
- more obvious the fatter you are
- swellings soft and not tender

Do you take any medication or drugs regularly?

no / yes

medication or drug side-effect
- non-medical, from cannabis
- if on medication, check the leaflet that comes with the tablets you take

Are you a heavy drinker or do you suffer from liver disease?

no / yes

liver disease
- in a drinker, a sign you have cirrhosis of the liver

Is one of your testicles enlarged and heavy?

no / yes

cancer of the testicle ⚠
- comes on gradually
- normally painless
- may also be some glands to feel in the groin

Only rare causes left, e.g.

cancer of the breast ⚠   **or thyroid problems**

Remember: ⚠ means see your GP sharpish; ⚠ means an urgent hospital job

Swelling of the breast

NB Yes, men do have breasts. Nothing that would ever appear on page three, admittedly, but they're there, right underneath your nipples.

Being overweight Flab can develop in all sorts of areas, including in the breasts. If you're really piling on the pounds, it is quite possible to develop fairly impressive bazookas.

Treatment Lose that lard – this means a sensible diet and more exercise. For more details, see the 'Middle-aged spread' part of the 'Weight gain' section (p. 153).

Puberty The hormonal turmoil that is puberty quite often makes one or both breasts swell for a while.

Treatment You're probably well beyond puberty by now and so can forget this as a cause. If you're not, then ignore your swellings if you can – you've got enough to worry about with other bits of your anatomy growing, sprouting, and erupting. You are definitely not turning into a woman and you'll find your boobs will disappear in time.

Medication or drug side-effect Some prescribed and over-the-counter medicines (including some strong indigestion cures) can cause minor changes in your hormones, resulting in breast growth. Cannabis can very occasionally have the same effect.

Treatment Either ignore the problem, as it's harmless, or stop whatever is causing it.

Liver disease Any long-term liver disease can affect the way your hormones work, leading to growth of your breast tissue with noticeable swellings. The most common cause in blokes is, by a long way, alcoholism.

Treatment The cure lies in stopping the booze. If you're drinking enough to cause liver damage then you're in serious trouble. You need to see your GP for a check-up and for help in kicking the habit.

Cancer of the testicle These cancers sometimes produce hormones which can make the breasts grow. They are explained in the 'Swelling in the scrotum' section (p. 132).

Breast cancer This is very nasty and, thankfully, incredibly rare in men.

Treatment See your GP asap – but you're much more likely to leave with reassurance than some bad news.

Other rare disorders Various other medical problems can occasionally show themselves by causing breast swelling, including lung cancer and thyroid problems.

Treatment If you think you have some problem which doesn't fit any of the categories already outlined above, see your GP.

Swelling on/around the face

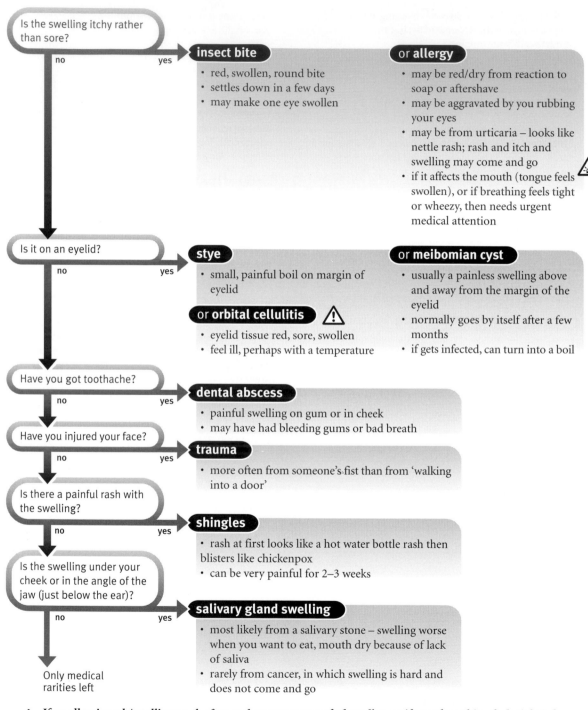

Is the swelling itchy rather than sore? — no / yes

insect bite
- red, swollen, round bite
- settles down in a few days
- may make one eye swollen

or allergy
- may be red/dry from reaction to soap or aftershave
- may be aggravated by you rubbing your eyes
- may be from urticaria – looks like nettle rash; rash and itch and swelling may come and go
- if it affects the mouth (tongue feels swollen), or if breathing feels tight or wheezy, then needs urgent medical attention

Is it on an eyelid? — no / yes

stye
- small, painful boil on margin of eyelid

or orbital cellulitis
- eyelid tissue red, sore, swollen
- feel ill, perhaps with a temperature

or meibomian cyst
- usually a painless swelling above and away from the margin of the eyelid
- normally goes by itself after a few months
- if gets infected, can turn into a boil

Have you got toothache? — no / yes

dental abscess
- painful swelling on gum or in cheek
- may have had bleeding gums or bad breath

Have you injured your face? — no / yes

trauma
- more often from someone's fist than from 'walking into a door'

Is there a painful rash with the swelling? — no / yes

shingles
- rash at first looks like a hot water bottle rash then blisters like chickenpox
- can be very painful for 2–3 weeks

Is the swelling under your cheek or in the angle of the jaw (just below the ear)? — no / yes

salivary gland swelling
- most likely from a salivary stone – swelling worse when you want to eat, mouth dry because of lack of saliva
- rarely from cancer, in which swelling is hard and does not come and go

Only medical rarities left

⚠ **If an allergic rash/swelling on the face makes your tongue feel swollen, or if your breathing feels tight/wheezy, seek medical attention urgently.**

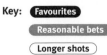
Insect bite Because the skin around the eye is quite slack, it can swell impressively after an insect bite.

Treatment It'll go on its own after a day or so. An ice-pack or antihistamine tablets (like you'd use for hay fever – available from the chemist) will help.

Stye This is an infection of the eyelid – the germ gets in around an eyelash, making the lid swollen and painful.

Treatment It'll sort itself out in a few days. Plucking out the eyelash in the centre of the stye may help. If the whole eye is getting red and sticky, you're probably developing conjunctivitis – try gently bathing the eye for a couple of days, but if it persists, see your GP for some antibiotic ointment.

Meibomian cyst If one of the tiny glands in your eyelid ('meibomian' glands) gets blocked, you end up with a pea-sized lump. This is common and harmless.

Treatment This can be left alone – it may eventually disappear on its own. If it doesn't and it's a nuisance, it can be cured with a very small operation: your GP can arrange this for you by referring you to an ophthalmologist (an eye specialist).

Trauma You don't have to be a rocket scientist to work out that a bash in the face might cause swelling.

Treatment If you've had a significant bump – say a punch or an elbow in the face – causing swelling, you need to go to casualty for an X-ray, as you may have a fracture.

Dental abscess This is an infection of the root of a tooth. The germ gets into the gum, making it swell.

Treatment You'll need some antibiotics and painkillers, so get to a dentist asap.

Allergy Two types of allergy can make your face swell. One is caused by something which has been in contact with your face, such as soap or shampoo. This tends to make the skin swell slightly and get itchy or sore, and is known as 'allergic contact eczema'. The other (called 'angio-oedema') results from a severe allergy to something which gets into your system. It has various causes, including foods, medications, and insects bites or stings – the reaction can be quite severe, so that your lips, tongue, or even your throat swell. In both types, you may previously have had no problems with whatever it is you've now developed an allergy to – it doesn't have to be something which is completely 'new' to you.

Treatment Treat allergic contact eczema with hydrocortisone 1% cream (available over the counter) and by avoiding whatever has caused it. Angio-oedema can get quite nasty, so you'll need to see your GP urgently for advice and treatment. Very rarely, the swelling can block your windpipe, so if you're having difficulty breathing, you need to go straight to hospital. Once you've been sorted out, you need to look at ways of preventing future attacks. Try to figure out what caused it, and be careful as far as possible to steer well clear of what you're allergic to in the future. Keep some antihistamines handy (available from the chemist) to use at the first sign of any trouble – they may nip another attack in the bud. If it turns out you've got a really severe allergy – to nuts or wasp stings for example – you may be given adrenaline (in the form of an injection) to use in case of future problems. Make sure you, and your nearest and dearest, know how to use it.

Shingles This is explained, and the treatment discussed, in the 'Blisters' section. If it occurs on the face, it can cause swelling on one side, especially on or around the eyelid – even before the blisters of shingles appear.

Orbital cellulitis See the 'Red eye' section (p. 121).

Salivary gland swellings The salivary glands produce the saliva which lubricates food when you chew. They are found just below your ear (parotid glands) and under your jaw (submandibular glands). They can swell for a number of reasons, including infections (such as mumps, although this is unusual nowadays) and stones (gravelly bits which block the tubes carrying the saliva). Very rarely, a persistent swelling of the parotid gland is caused by a growth.

Treatment This depends on the cause. Many of the infections are caused by viruses and go away on their own. Other types may need antibiotics, so if the swelling is very sore, showing no signs of going down, or you feel ill or feverish, see your GP. Swellings caused by stones can be cured by stimulating the flow of saliva (with lemon drops, for example) or with a small operation. Growths need sorting out by a specialist.

Medical rarities A few small print problems can make the face puff up (such as an underactive thyroid gland or the side-effects of steroid treatment) or cause an obviously swollen area (such as bone or sinus cancer).

Treatment These are very unlikely to be the cause of your problem. If you're concerned, discuss the situation with your GP.

Swollen glands

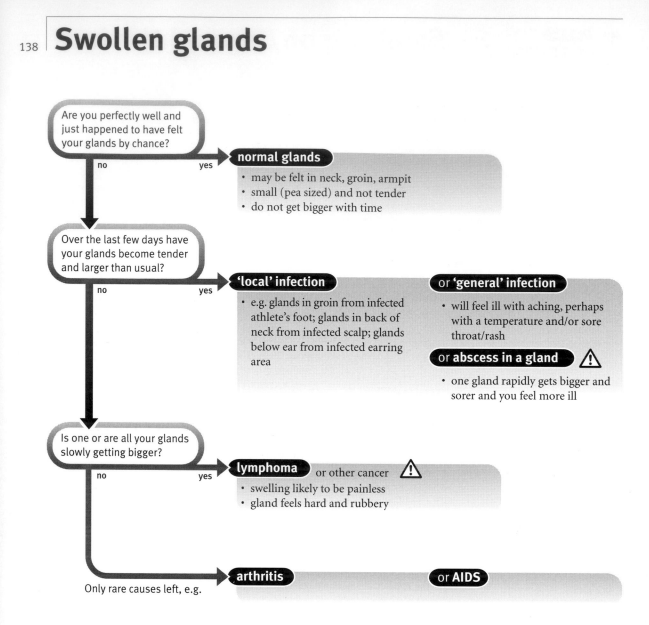

Are you perfectly well and just happened to have felt your glands by chance?

no   yes

normal glands
- may be felt in neck, groin, armpit
- small (pea sized) and not tender
- do not get bigger with time

Over the last few days have your glands become tender and larger than usual?

no   yes

'local' infection
- e.g. glands in groin from infected athlete's foot; glands in back of neck from infected scalp; glands below ear from infected earring area

or 'general' infection
- will feel ill with aching, perhaps with a temperature and/or sore throat/rash

or abscess in a gland ⚠
- one gland rapidly gets bigger and sorer and you feel more ill

Is one or are all your glands slowly getting bigger?

no   yes

lymphoma or other cancer ⚠
- swelling likely to be painless
- gland feels hard and rubbery

Only rare causes left, e.g.

arthritis   or **AIDS**

Remember: ⚠ means see your GP sharpish; ⚠ means an urgent hospital job

Swollen glands

Normal glands Glands are found in various parts of the body – particularly the neck, the armpits, and the groin. They are a part of your immune system, which helps fight off infections. If you're slim, it's quite normal to be able to feel these glands as pea-sized, non-tender lumps which stay roughly the same size most of the time.

Treatment Being able to feel these glands is entirely normal, so no treatment is needed.

'Local' infection If a germ gets into one part of your body, the glands nearby will swell as they try to fight it off. For example, your neck glands will enlarge if you get a sore throat, and the glands in your groin may swell if you pick up a sexually transmitted germ.

Treatment The glands themselves don't need any treatment – the fact that they've swollen just means they're doing their job. But the infection which has made them swell may need sorting out. So unless it's just a case of your neck glands swelling up a bit with a mild sore throat, see your GP.

'General' infection Some germs don't stick in one area – instead they get right into your system, making all your glands swell up. Examples include viruses like glandular fever and German measles (rare nowadays, as all children are immunized against this).

Treatment Again, the glands themselves don't need treating. The fact that they've swollen means they're trying to fight off the germ. In fact, because most of these infections are caused by viruses, there's usually no magic cure – you simply have to wait for them to burn themselves out. Paracetamol will help the fever, aches and pains, and sore throat which often go with this type of problem; for more information on treating glandular fever, see the 'Sore throat' section. If you feel very ill and feverish, you ought to discuss the situation with your GP.

Abscess in a gland If a particular type of germ gets into a gland, it can sometimes produce a large boil-like swelling, full of pus. This is an abscess.

Treatment If it's only just come on, antibiotics may cure it. But if it's developed into a full-blown abscess, it'll need lancing to let the pus out. Either way, you'll need to see your GP.

Lymphoma This is a cancer of the lymph glands.

Treatment It's unlikely that this is the cause of your problem, but, if you're worried it could be, you obviously need to see your GP asap. If he shares your concern, he'll probably run some tests and refer you to a specialist. The treatment is unpleasant – chemotherapy (powerful drugs) or radiotherapy (radiation beam treatment) – but offers a chance of cure.

Other rare medical conditions Lots of other rarities can make the glands of the body swell. These include some types of arthritis, other cancers, AIDS, and the side-effects of some medication.

Treatment See your GP if you're worried that you might have one of these unusual causes. He'll arrange any necessary tests and treatment.

Tired all the time

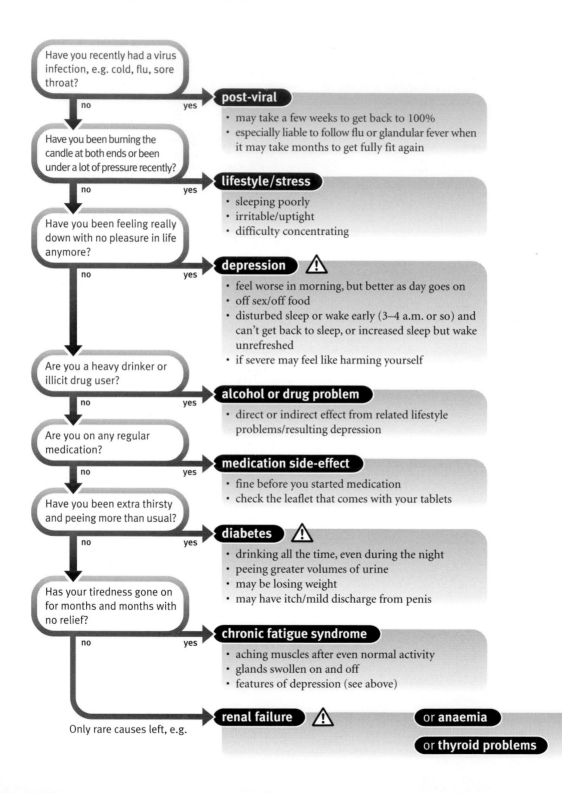

Have you recently had a virus infection, e.g. cold, flu, sore throat?

no / **yes**

post-viral
- may take a few weeks to get back to 100%
- especially liable to follow flu or glandular fever when it may take months to get fully fit again

Have you been burning the candle at both ends or been under a lot of pressure recently?

no / **yes**

lifestyle/stress
- sleeping poorly
- irritable/uptight
- difficulty concentrating

Have you been feeling really down with no pleasure in life anymore?

no / **yes**

depression
- feel worse in morning, but better as day goes on
- off sex/off food
- disturbed sleep or wake early (3–4 a.m. or so) and can't get back to sleep, or increased sleep but wake unrefreshed
- if severe may feel like harming yourself

Are you a heavy drinker or illicit drug user?

no / **yes**

alcohol or drug problem
- direct or indirect effect from related lifestyle problems/resulting depression

Are you on any regular medication?

no / **yes**

medication side-effect
- fine before you started medication
- check the leaflet that comes with your tablets

Have you been extra thirsty and peeing more than usual?

no / **yes**

diabetes
- drinking all the time, even during the night
- peeing greater volumes of urine
- may be losing weight
- may have itch/mild discharge from penis

Has your tiredness gone on for months and months with no relief?

no / **yes**

chronic fatigue syndrome
- aching muscles after even normal activity
- glands swollen on and off
- features of depression (see above)

Only rare causes left, e.g.

renal failure **or anaemia** **or thyroid problems**

Lifestyle/stress Tiredness is one of the complaints your GP deals with daily. If there are no other particular symptoms, such as weight loss, it's very unlikely to be caused by a disease. In fact, research has shown that, when questioned, up to a third of people feel 'tired all the time'. In most cases, there isn't one specific cause – the tiredness is due to a mixture of things such as poor or irregular sleep, lack of physical exercise, and pressure at work. Stress usually plays a part: it's exhausting being uptight all the time.

Treatment There's no magic pill, so don't bother your chemist or doctor. A sensible approach is to take a long hard look at your lifestyle and make some constructive changes. It's important to sort out your sleeping habits: go to bed at a set time as far as possible and try to get more sleep, but avoid daytime naps and lying in. You'll sleep – and feel – better if you increase the amount of physical exercise you take. Try to sort out any sources of stress in your life and wind down with some relaxation therapy (see the 'Feeling tense' section).

Post-viral Any recent virus – especially influenza and glandular fever – can leave you feeling below par for some weeks. This is particularly the case if your lifestyle isn't particularly restful or you've made a very quick return to work.

Treatment There is no specific treatment for this – you simply have to be patient and try some of the measures outlined above while you wait for your energy levels to return to normal.

Depression This is explained, and its treatment outlined, in the 'Feeling down' section (p. 57).

Alcohol or drug problem Alcohol or drugs can cause tiredness in a number of ways. They can directly sap energy levels; they can make your life chaotic, resulting in a poor diet, no exercise, and a lack of sleep; and they can cause depression.

Treatment Cut down – or better still, stop – the substance abuse and get a grip on your lifestyle. If you find it difficult and want help, check out your local drug or alcohol services (try the Citizen's Advice Bureau or the 'phone directory) or see your GP.

Medication side-effect Some prescribed treatments, such as pills for blood pressure or antidepressants, can cause tiredness as a side-effect.

Treatment Check the leaflet in the treatment pack, or ask your pharmacist to see if tiredness is a side-effect of any medication you're taking. If it is, then speak to your GP. It can be difficult to know whether or not to blame the treatment, as tiredness is so common anyway, whether people are on medication or not. If your GP thinks your medica-

tion could be the cause, then he may be able to stop it or switch you to an alternative.

Diabetes This is explained, and the treatment described, in the 'Impotence' section (p. 69).

Chronic fatigue syndrome This is known by a variety of other names – in the past, 'Yuppy flu' and, more recently, 'ME' (short for myalgic encephalomyelitis). Chronic fatigue syndrome (CFS), meaning 'long-term tiredness', is widely regarded as a better name, but this is where the agreement ends and the controversy begins. Pages have been written in the tabloids, the broadsheets, and the learned medical journals, but there's still a lot of debate about what CFS is exactly and what causes it. Some heated arguments have raged about whether the problem is in the mind or body, but most doctors now agree it's probably a bit of both. CFS is a feeling of severe tiredness which won't go away and which may be linked with aching muscles, swollen glands, and feelings of depression. No one is sure what triggers it – it may be a virus, an emotional upset, or something else. Nor does anyone know what keeps it going, although psychological factors are thought to play a part. These might include a negative or pessimistic attitude, an incorrect belief that 'a virus' is still lurking in the body, and an unwillingness to try even small amounts of exercise. In the worst cases, people can become very disabled and the symptoms can go on for years.

Treatment As no one can agree on what causes CFS, it's no surprise that the treatment depends very much on who you listen to. There is certainly no magic pill to sort out the problem. Doctors who've done a lot of research into CFS believe it's very important to take a positive approach and to avoid looking for miracle cures – there are plenty of quack treatments around, but they're not based on scientific fact and they may burn a hole in your wallet. Gentle exercise, gradually increased, is likely to help. It's important not to overdo it at first, otherwise the resulting exhaustion will make you want to 'give up', so you'll be one step forwards and two back, and prone to developing a 'can't do' attitude. Antidepressants help some patients if feeling down is a big part of the problem. Your best bet is to discuss the situation with your GP. Try not to be too up front with your self-diagnosis, as your doc will have encountered many before you who were convinced they had 'ME' but turned out to have some other problem.

Other medical problems Tiredness can be a feature of a huge range of medical problems such as anaemia, thyroid trouble, and kidney failure. It's pretty unlikely you'll have any of these.

Treatment See your GP, who'll arrange the necessary tests if he's concerned.

Tremor

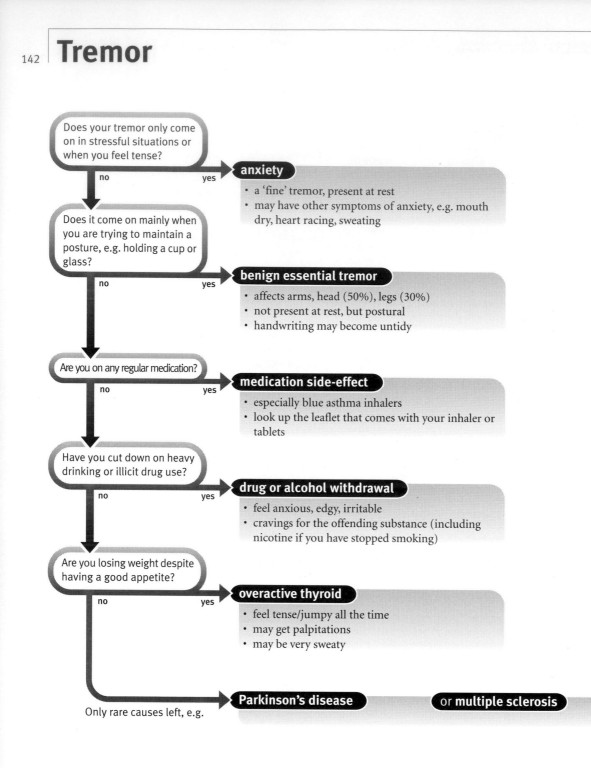

Does your tremor only come on in stressful situations or when you feel tense?

no / yes

anxiety
- a 'fine' tremor, present at rest
- may have other symptoms of anxiety, e.g. mouth dry, heart racing, sweating

Does it come on mainly when you are trying to maintain a posture, e.g. holding a cup or glass?

no / yes

benign essential tremor
- affects arms, head (50%), legs (30%)
- not present at rest, but postural
- handwriting may become untidy

Are you on any regular medication?

no / yes

medication side-effect
- especially blue asthma inhalers
- look up the leaflet that comes with your inhaler or tablets

Have you cut down on heavy drinking or illicit drug use?

no / yes

drug or alcohol withdrawal
- feel anxious, edgy, irritable
- cravings for the offending substance (including nicotine if you have stopped smoking)

Are you losing weight despite having a good appetite?

no / yes

overactive thyroid
- feel tense/jumpy all the time
- may get palpitations
- may be very sweaty

Only rare causes left, e.g.

Parkinson's disease   or **multiple sclerosis**

Anxiety If you're frightened or angry, you'll know it's normal to tremble. This can happen constantly if you're feeling very tense all the time, or, occasionally, if you get really anxious in certain situations.

Treatment The treatment of anxiety is discussed in the 'Palpitations' (p. 103) and 'Feeling tense' (p. 59) sections – exactly the same principles apply with tremor. If the tremor is a real problem – particularly if it affects your performance when you get uptight doing, for example, a speech or a presentation – your GP may be able to give you some tablets to ease it.

Benign essential tremor Everyone experiences a tremor, but most aren't aware of it because it's very slight (you can prove this by putting a piece of A4 paper over your outstretched hand – you'll see the edges of the paper shake). In some people, for some reason, this normal tremor is much more obvious – this is called benign essential tremor. It often runs in families.

Treatment This is harmless and will not develop into anything more serious, so it's safe to leave it alone. You'll probably find that a small alcoholic drink gets rid of the problem completely for a short period of time, though, for obvious reasons, this can't be recommended as a regular treatment. If the tremor is a real nuisance, discuss it with your GP. He might prescribe some tablets which can help ease the problem.

Medication side-effect Some prescribed treatments, such as drugs for severe psychiatric conditions, can cause tremor as a side-effect. It can also be caused by certain asthma inhalers (the 'treater' inhalers, such as salbutamol and terbutaline), especially if you're using them too much.

Treatment If you think your medication might be causing a tremor, discuss the situation with your GP. When the tremor is caused by overuse of asthma inhalers, you obviously need to ease up on them and you may need to see your GP – using too many inhalers probably means that your asthma isn't under proper control, so the doc may want to alter your treatment. Of course, if you've been bashing the inhalers because you're having a bad asthma attack, you need to see your GP urgently.

Drug or alcohol withdrawal If your body has been used to regular doses of a drug or alcohol which is suddenly stopped, you may suffer a 'withdrawal syndrome' – symptoms caused by the body craving the drug. Most people are familiar with this happening with illegal addictive drugs, but it can also be caused by suddenly stopping alcohol and some prescribed treatments. A tremor is one of the signs of drug withdrawal.

Treatment If the tremor isn't too bad, and other symptoms of withdrawal aren't a great problem, then just sit it out – it'll settle down in due course. But if the withdrawal syndrome is giving you real problems, seek help via your GP or the local drug or alcohol unit. You'll probably be given some medication as a 'substitute' for whatever your body is craving, and then weaned off this treatment slowly so you don't suffer bad withdrawal effects.

Overactive thyroid This is explained, and its treatment outlined, in the 'Excess sweating' section (p. 55).

Rare medical causes Diseases of the nervous system (such as Parkinson's disease or multiple sclerosis) can cause a tremor. But they're either very rare in men under 50, or are likely to be causing other, more worrying, symptoms than tremor and so are very unlikely to be the cause.

Treatment See your GP. If he shares your concerns, he'll refer you to a neurologist (a nervous system specialist) for further tests.

Vision problems

(If you have a Red eye see p. 120)

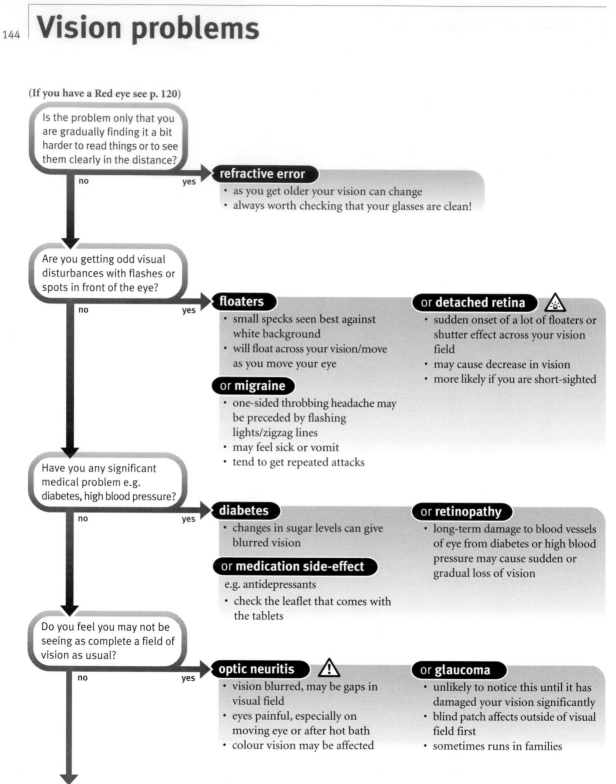

Is the problem only that you are gradually finding it a bit harder to read things or to see them clearly in the distance?

no — yes

refractive error
- as you get older your vision can change
- always worth checking that your glasses are clean!

Are you getting odd visual disturbances with flashes or spots in front of the eye?

no — yes

floaters
- small specks seen best against white background
- will float across your vision/move as you move your eye

or detached retina
- sudden onset of a lot of floaters or shutter effect across your vision field
- may cause decrease in vision
- more likely if you are short-sighted

or migraine
- one-sided throbbing headache may be preceded by flashing lights/zigzag lines
- may feel sick or vomit
- tend to get repeated attacks

Have you any significant medical problem e.g. diabetes, high blood pressure?

no — yes

diabetes
- changes in sugar levels can give blurred vision

or retinopathy
- long-term damage to blood vessels of eye from diabetes or high blood pressure may cause sudden or gradual loss of vision

or medication side-effect
e.g. antidepressants
- check the leaflet that comes with the tablets

Do you feel you may not be seeing as complete a field of vision as usual?

no — yes

optic neuritis
- vision blurred, may be gaps in visual field
- eyes painful, especially on moving eye or after hot bath
- colour vision may be affected

or glaucoma
- unlikely to notice this until it has damaged your vision significantly
- blind patch affects outside of visual field first
- sometimes runs in families

Only other rare causes left

If you get a sudden onset of flashers/floaters, especially with decreased vision, or if you get a sudden loss of all or part of your field of vision, seek medical attention urgently.

Vision problems

Refractive errors The eye is like a camera. The iris (the coloured part of your eye) is the aperture, letting the light in. It's focused by the lens and the cornea (the clear part of the front of the eye) onto the retina at the back of the eye – the equivalent of the film. Problems with the cornea, lens, or shape of the eye which stop the light from focusing on the retina properly are called 'refractive errors'. These include: short-sightedness, when you can see clearly close up but not in the distance; long-sightedness, when the reverse applies; and astigmatism, when the cornea is uneven causing blurring for far and near vision.

Treatment You don't need to do anything about it if it doesn't bother you – but make sure your eyesight is still OK for you to drive. If you want to sort it out, see your optician, who will be able to arrange glasses or contact lenses for you. You can also consider surgery which alters the curve of your cornea and so improves your vision. But bear in mind that the results aren't always fantastic, there can be side-effects, and it's only available privately, so you're likely to have to fork out loads of money.

Floaters Bits of debris can collect together inside the eye. These float around in the fluid inside the eyeball and are seen – particularly against a white background – as small specks or spidery shadows.

Treatment These can be a nuisance but are harmless. There's no treatment and they're usually permanent, although you get used to them so they become less noticeable in time. Very occasionally they can be a sign of a 'detached retina' (see 'Other rare medical problems' below), in which case they come on suddenly in a 'shower', usually with blurred vision. This needs assessment by your doc urgently.

Migraine If you get migraine, your eyesight may be affected before the headache comes on. This is because migraine starts with a tightening up of blood vessels to your brain, which can result in the part dealing with your vision being starved of oxygen for a short while. This can cause blurring, flashing lights, or tunnel vision. For further information about migraine, see the 'Headache' section (p. 63).

Diabetes This is explained in the 'Impotence' section (p. 69). The high blood sugar in your bloodstream can lead to your vision blurring. Diabetes can also cause 'retinopathy' (see below).

Treatment See the 'Impotence' section. If you're a 'known' diabetic, keep a close eye on your sugar readings and adjust your treatment if necessary and you're confident you know what to do – if not, contact your GP or the local diabetes nurse.

Retinopathy This means a disease of the retina. The commonest causes are high blood pressure and diabetes. They may cause more dramatic problems with vision such as sudden complete or partial blindness, but they may also result in gradual blurring.

Treatment See your GP to get the cause diagnosed and treated. This problem is sometimes picked up by your optician, who will then send you on to your doctor.

Medication side-effect Some prescribed medications, such as antidepressants, can affect the way your eye focuses, leading to blurred vision.

Treatment The problem will often correct itself as your body gets used to the treatment, so persevere for a while if you can. If it doesn't, speak to your GP – he may be able to stop the medication, or swap it for something else.

Optic neuritis This is an inflammation of the nerve which supplies the retina. Some attacks are thought to be caused by a virus. Others are a part of – or the first sign of – multiple sclerosis (explained further in the 'Pins and needles and numbness' section).

Treatment See your GP asap. If you're known to have multiple sclerosis, he may let the problem settle on its own or he may prescribe you steroid tablets. Otherwise, he'll probably just keep an eye on the situation, as most attacks – especially those caused by viruses – go away on their own, although you may be left with some slight blurring or dimming of your vision (especially for colours). But if your doctor suspects you might be developing multiple sclerosis, he'll refer you to a neurologist (a nerve specialist).

Glaucoma If the pressure of the fluid in your eye is too high, it can damage the retina. This problem sometimes runs in families. You're unlikely to notice it, especially at first, because it tends to affect only how well you see out of the corners of your eyes. It's more likely to be spotted during a routine check by your optician.

Treatment Your optician will give you a letter to take to your GP, who will then probably refer you to an eye specialist for a thorough check and, if necessary, treatment. If you have a family history of glaucoma but don't have any problem yourself, it's important to get regular eye checks from your optician.

Other rare medical problems A variety of small print problems can blur your vision, including a detached retina, rare infections, and brain tumours.

Treatment It's highly unlikely you'll have any of these problems. If you're concerned, speak to your GP.

Vomiting

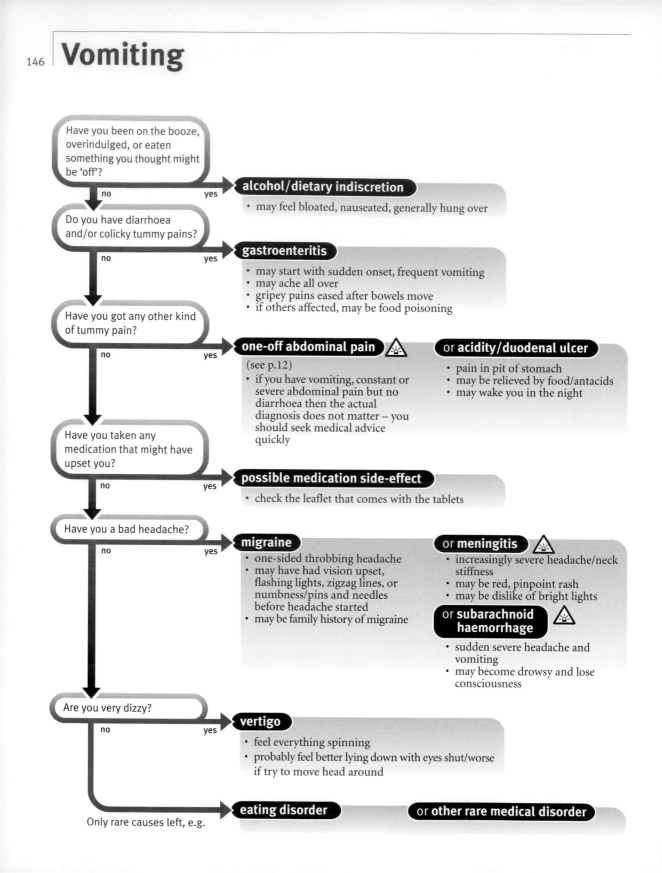

Have you been on the booze, overindulged, or eaten something you thought might be 'off'?

no / yes

alcohol/dietary indiscretion
- may feel bloated, nauseated, generally hung over

Do you have diarrhoea and/or colicky tummy pains?

no / yes

gastroenteritis
- may start with sudden onset, frequent vomiting
- may ache all over
- gripey pains eased after bowels move
- if others affected, may be food poisoning

Have you got any other kind of tummy pain?

no / yes

one-off abdominal pain
(see p.12)
- if you have vomiting, constant or severe abdominal pain but no diarrhoea then the actual diagnosis does not matter – you should seek medical advice quickly

or acidity/duodenal ulcer
- pain in pit of stomach
- may be relieved by food/antacids
- may wake you in the night

Have you taken any medication that might have upset you?

no / yes

possible medication side-effect
- check the leaflet that comes with the tablets

Have you a bad headache?

no / yes

migraine
- one-sided throbbing headache
- may have had vision upset, flashing lights, zigzag lines, or numbness/pins and needles before headache started
- may be family history of migraine

or meningitis
- increasingly severe headache/neck stiffness
- may be red, pinpoint rash
- may be dislike of bright lights

or subarachnoid haemorrhage
- sudden severe headache and vomiting
- may become drowsy and lose consciousness

Are you very dizzy?

no / yes

vertigo
- feel everything spinning
- probably feel better lying down with eyes shut/worse if try to move head around

eating disorder

or other rare medical disorder

Only rare causes left, e.g.

⚠️ If you have vomiting with sudden severe headache/pain in the back of your neck, or increasing headache and neck stiffness, seek medical help immediately to exclude subarachnoid haemorrhage or meningitis.

⚠️ If you have vomiting with abdominal pain (not gripey with diarrhoea) then there may be a serious cause and you must seek medical advice immediately.

Alcohol/dietary indiscretion Vomiting after, say, 10 pints of lager and a vindaloo is your stomach's way of saying, 'Thanks, but no thanks' – or of making room for more, depending on how you look at it.

Treatment This is an unpleasant but perfectly normal reaction, and so needs no specific treatment. You may want to treat the hangover the following morning, though: plenty of non-alcoholic fluids, painkillers for the headache, and antacids for any gut rot. And as regards prevention – it's simply a case of being more sensible on the booze and biriani front in future.

Gastroenteritis This is explained, and the treatment outlined, in the 'Abdominal pain – one-off' section (p. 13).

One-off abdominal pain Many causes of severe belly ache produce vomiting, including appendicitis, ulcers, renal colic, gallstones, pancreatitis, and bowel obstruction. For more details, see the 'Abdominal pain – one-off' section.

Medication side-effect Lots of different medications can irritate the stomach, leading to vomiting. Examples include anti-inflammatory drugs (such as ibuprofen) and antibiotics. Powerful drugs for cancers (known as 'chemotherapy') can cause severe vomiting, but if you're unlucky enough to be on this type of treatment, you'll have been warned about this side-effect – and you'll probably have been prescribed something to counteract it.

Treatment If the offending treatment was prescribed by your doc, discuss the situation with him. But if you bought the treatment over the counter, either simply stop it or have a word with your chemist.

Migraine This is explained, and the treatment outlined, in the 'Headache' section (p. 63).

Vertigo Many causes of vertigo (a feeling of unsteadiness or of the world spinning around) can lead to vomiting. The problem is explained fully, and treatment discussed, in the 'Dizziness' section (p. 49).

(**Acidity/duodenal ulcer**) This can show itself with a 'bang', causing severe belly pain, or it can grumble off and on for some time – more details, and advice about treatment, are given in the 'Abdominal pain – one-off' section (p. 13). Bad bouts can inflame the stomach lining so badly that you end up with repeated bouts of vomiting.

(**Eating disorder**) This is explained, and the treatment discussed, in the 'Weight loss' section (p. 155). Vomiting is usually 'self-induced' – a finger down the throat job.

(**Rare and serious medical problems**) There are huge numbers of pretty nasty medical conditions which can cause vomiting – but they usually come to light through other symptoms. They include meningitis, subarachnoid haemorrhage and brain tumours (see 'Headache' section, p. 63), kidney failure, and stomach cancer.

Treatment It's very unlikely that you'll have any of these problems. Meningitis and subarachnoid haemorrhage require the services of an urgent ambulance. For anything else, you need to see your GP asap.

Vomiting up blood

⚠ Regardless of the possible cause, if you vomit up more than a cupful of blood, vomit up blood more than once, or feel faint or ill as well, then go to hospital without delay. Note also: vomited blood can look like 'coffee grounds'.

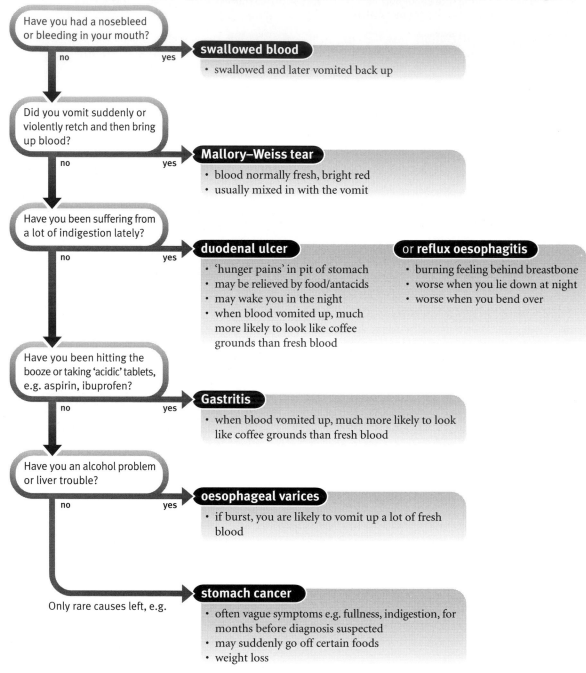

Have you had a nosebleed or bleeding in your mouth?

no / yes

swallowed blood
- swallowed and later vomited back up

Did you vomit suddenly or violently retch and then bring up blood?

no / yes

Mallory–Weiss tear
- blood normally fresh, bright red
- usually mixed in with the vomit

Have you been suffering from a lot of indigestion lately?

no / yes

duodenal ulcer
- 'hunger pains' in pit of stomach
- may be relieved by food/antacids
- may wake you in the night
- when blood vomited up, much more likely to look like coffee grounds than fresh blood

or reflux oesophagitis
- burning feeling behind breastbone
- worse when you lie down at night
- worse when you bend over

Have you been hitting the booze or taking 'acidic' tablets, e.g. aspirin, ibuprofen?

no / yes

Gastritis
- when blood vomited up, much more likely to look like coffee grounds than fresh blood

Have you an alcohol problem or liver trouble?

no / yes

oesophageal varices
- if burst, you are likely to vomit up a lot of fresh blood

Only rare causes left, e.g.

stomach cancer
- often vague symptoms e.g. fullness, indigestion, for months before diagnosis suspected
- may suddenly go off certain foods
- weight loss

Vomiting up blood

Swallowed blood Blood from a nosebleed, or, less commonly, blood coughed up from the lungs, can be swallowed and then vomited back up again.

Treatment If it's obviously blood you've swallowed from a nosebleed, then you have nothing to worry about. If it's blood you've been coughing up, then you need to look at the 'Blood in Spit' flow chart (p. 34).

Mallory–Weiss tear A violent retch during vomiting can tear a blood vessel in the stomach or gullet, causing leakage of blood. This is then brought up in the next vomit.

Treatment If it's a small amount of blood (say less than a cupful) mixed in with the vomit, and it happens only once, and you otherwise feel reasonably OK (apart from the vomiting, of course), then there's nothing to worry about. But if it's more than this, it keeps happening, or you feel very ill, then you could have lost a significant amount of blood. Your best bet is to go to casualty, pronto.

Gastritis Overdoing the booze (especially binge drinking), or using a lot of 'acidic' tablets like ibuprofen or aspirin, can inflame the stomach lining. This is called gastritis, and it can cause bleeding, just like it does in reflux oesophagitis (see below).

Treatment You'll need checking over at the hospital and will probably be given a course of acid-suppressant treatment – and, in the future, you'll need to avoid whatever brought it on in the first place.

Duodenal ulcer This is explained in the 'Acidity/duodenal ulcer' part of the 'Abdominal pain – recurrent' section (p. 15) and also the 'Duodenal or gastric ulcer' part of the 'Indigestion' section (p. 71). A duodenal ulcer can bleed, leading to blood being vomited – or the blood may appear in your motions as 'melaena' (black, tarry, very smelly motions, which are partially digested blood). The problem may be caused or aggravated by some 'insult' to your guts – such as an alcoholic binge or taking acidic tablets like ibuprofen.

Treatment These types of bleeds are usually bad enough to need hospital treatment. You may well end up on acid-suppressant drugs for life. For other measures you can take to prevent trouble in the future, see the 'Abdominal pain – recurrent' (p. 15) and 'Indigestion' (p. 71) sections.

Reflux oesophagitis This is explained in the 'Indigestion' section (p. 71). If the lining of the gullet gets very inflamed, it may leak blood, which can be vomited up. It can pass out the other end, too, as 'melaena' (see above).

Treatment You're likely to need hospital tests and treatment, so go to casualty. Once sorted out, you can then look at a number of areas you can tweak to try to prevent trouble in the future – these are explained in the 'Indigestion' section (p. 71). If you've had a serious bleed caused by reflux oesophagitis, then you may be put on an acid-suppressant drug indefinitely.

Oesophageal varices These are huge varicose veins – bloated blood vessels – in your gullet. When one pops, it causes dramatic bleeding.

Treatment There won't be much doubt about what to do in this situation: get an ambulance.

Other rare problems There are a few medical rarities which might cause this symptom, such as stomach cancer. The cancer can eat its way into a blood vessel; the leaked blood is then vomited up. Thankfully, this is very, very unlikely in men under the age of 50.

Treatment Most rare problems are likely to cause a lot of blood in the vomit, so hospital treatment is needed urgently. If the blood is only a small amount and only happens from time to time, consult your doctor.

Waterworks problems

Are you really uptight or very worried about something?

no — yes →

anxiety

- irritable/tense
- either difficulty getting off to sleep or restless/ fragmented sleep as you wake in night worrying
- once you start worrying that you are peeing too much then this will make the problem appear worse (start noticing every time you blink and you will see what we mean)

Do your symptoms seem to be mainly at night or worse at night?

no — yes →

alcohol related

- unless you are so pissed you don't even wake up to pee, drinking in the evening will have you up in the night peeing

or diabetes ⚠

- wake to pee and drink as so thirsty
- may be losing weight
- may have itch/mild discharge from penis

or prostate enlargement

- often, first sign is waking to pee
- may notice bit of difficulty starting to pee/not such a strong flow/bit of dribbling at end

Is there any risk you could have caught a sexually transmitted disease?

no — yes →

urethritis

- stinging when you pee
- discharge from penis

Does it sting when you pee?

no — yes →

prostatitis

- may be pain or ache just behind the penis or up your bottom
- may be ache or stinging when you pee
- may cause blood in sperm

or urinary tract infection

- if in bladder, get burning, urgency (must go as soon as you get urge), and perhaps blood in urine
- if in kidney, may get high temperature, pain over kidney area

Only rare causes left, e.g.

urethral stricture

- perhaps from previous attacks of urethritis
- urine may spray all over the place and stream is weak

or unstable bladder

or medication side-effect

- perhaps from water tablets sometimes used to treat high blood pressure

or bladder stone

Anxiety The bladder is a muscular bag (like the bag inside a leather football) which collects your wee until you're ready to pass it. If you're uptight, the bladder tenses up, so it can't hold as much urine as usual. Being stressed also makes the bladder muscle twitchy, which will make you want to keep running to the loo. You'll have noticed this when you've felt nervous about something (like before an interview). The same thing can happen if you're very cold.

Treatment This is a normal reaction, so no treatment is needed. You might get persistent trouble if you're feeling anxious all the time – try the techniques explained in the 'Anxiety' part of the 'Feeling tense' (p. 59) and 'Palpitations' (p. 103) sections.

Urethritis This is explained, and its treatment outlined, in the 'Penis problems' section (p. 105).

Alcohol related Booze tends to get converted into large amounts of urine – which is why you may need several visits to the khazi during a session down the pub. This will affect some blokes more than others, as bladder capacities vary. A real binge can result in you wetting the bed – partly because your bladder can't cope with all the pee you've produced and partly because the alcohol makes you less aware of what you're doing.

Treatment Cut down on the booze if it's causing you a problem. Drinking shorts rather than beer or lager may help because the volume is smaller.

Prostatitis This is explained in the 'Blood in the sperm' section (p. 33). The infected prostate gland can make you pass water much more often and can make it uncomfortable too.

Treatment See the 'Blood in the sperm' section (p. 33).

Urinary tract infection (UTI) Germs can infect the bladder and kidneys, making you want to pass water very often and making you rush to the loo. A UTI will make it sting when you pee too – but, unlike urethritis, this type of infection isn't passed on by sex.

Treatment See your GP and take a specimen of urine with you for him to test. If you do have a UTI, he'll prescribe some antibiotics. You may also be referred to a hospital specialist for some tests, as it's quite unusual for blokes to get these infections – you've about a one in four chance of having some other problem which has brought it on, like a stone (see below).

Urethral stricture This is a narrowing of your urethra. It's usually caused by a previous injury or infection (especially urethritis).

Treatment See your GP if it's becoming a problem. A small operation to open up the urethra should sort it out, though it may have to be done again in the future.

(**Unstable bladder**) This means the bladder muscle works to empty the bladder when you're not expecting it, so you have to rush the loo, probably only to pee a small amount, and you might even wet yourself. It's much commoner in women than men.

Treatment Another GP job, again with a urine specimen for him to check out. If he thinks you might have an unstable bladder, he'll probably refer you to a specialist for further tests.

(**Bladder stone**) Stones – like bits of gravel – can form anywhere in the waterworks. A stone in the bladder will bounce about, making you want to keep peeing, and making you feel like you haven't emptied your bladder properly.

Treatment You'll be referred to a urologist (a waterworks specialist) to get this sorted out.

(**Medication side-effect**) Some prescribed treatments, such as antidepressants, can occasionally make it difficult to pee properly; others (commonly known as 'water tablets') make you pee more, though you're highly unlikely to be on these.

Treatment If you think your medication is upsetting your waterworks, see your GP.

(**Diabetes**) This is explained, and its treatment outlined, in the 'Impotence' section (p. 69).

(**Prostate enlargement**) The prostate gland is the size of a small walnut and sits at the base of the bladder, with the tube which carries urine (the urethra) going right through it. It produces some of the fluid which makes up sperm. It gets bigger as you get older ('benign hypertrophy') and can press on the bladder and squeeze the urethra, causing a variety of waterworks troubles. Occasionally, a swollen prostate is caused by prostate cancer.

Treatment Discuss the problem with your GP. He may be able to reassure you after a check-over and perhaps a blood test, or he may need to refer you to a urologist.

Weight gain

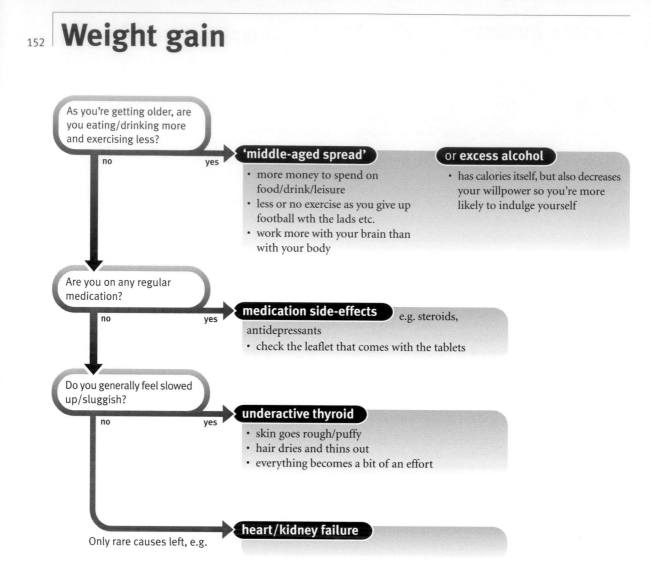

As you're getting older, are you eating/drinking more and exercising less?

no / yes

'middle-aged spread'
- more money to spend on food/drink/leisure
- less or no exercise as you give up football wth the lads etc.
- work more with your brain than with your body

or excess alcohol
- has calories itself, but also decreases your willpower so you're more likely to indulge yourself

Are you on any regular medication?

no / yes

medication side-effects e.g. steroids, antidepressants
- check the leaflet that comes with the tablets

Do you generally feel slowed up/sluggish?

no / yes

underactive thyroid
- skin goes rough/puffy
- hair dries and thins out
- everything becomes a bit of an effort

Only rare causes left, e.g.

heart/kidney failure

'Middle-aged spread' Far and away the commonest cause of weight gain is a lousy lifestyle which makes you put on fat. About 45% of men in this country are overweight. There's nothing complicated about working out how and why the weight goes on. If you take in more fuel (food and drink) than you burn off (in exercise) then the surplus is stored – in the form of fat. As you get older, your metabolism – the rate at which you use up the fuel – slows down. So, to keep the same weight, you need to eat less or exercise more. Usually, the opposite happens, so the dreaded middle-aged spread develops.

Treatment There's no easy answer, although thousands are advertised – most miracle cures are simply there to make a fast buck. The only effective way to sort out your weight in the long term is to alter your lifestyle – this means eating more healthily and taking more exercise. You don't need to go on a crash diet. Healthy eating is the rule with plenty of fruit, fresh vegetables, fibre, white meat, and fish rather than fast and junk foods, red meat, cakes, and so on – advice you're likely to have heard before. Sensible diet sheets are readily available at the chemist's and your doctor's. Aim for a steady weight loss and consider joining a group if you're very fat or having real problems shedding the lard. Exercise regularly and gradually build up the amount you do – use your common sense and don't go hell for leather from day one, as sudden and extreme exercise can be bad for the unfit body. There's very little point seeing your GP for a magic bullet, as drug treatment is not usually viewed as a sensible or effective way to slim down. He may be able to point you in the direction of a good diet or slimming group, and can advise you about exercise, though. And if you're only a few pounds overweight, don't get too obsessed about it as it probably isn't that bad for you – and you still need to enjoy life.

Excess alcohol Booze is full of calories – so if you've read the information about 'middle-aged spread', above, you'll be able to work out why drinking too much will pile on the weight. If you're developing a serious alcohol problem, you can end up seriously ill and retaining a lot of fluid, which will also make you gain weight.

Treatment Cut down your intake. And if you think you have a major problem, see your GP as you will need a careful check-up, advice on how to stop drinking and, maybe, the help of a specialist.

Medication side-effect Some treatments, such as antidepressants, migraine-preventers, and steroids, can cause weight gain as a side-effect. Anabolic steroids, as used by some body-builders, can cause the same problem.

Treatment Check the leaflet with your medication to see if weight gain is a side-effect. If so, discuss the situation with your GP.

Underactive thyroid The thyroid gland sits in the front of your neck and produces a hormone, 'thyroxine', which controls your metabolism. If it becomes underactive, it stops producing enough thyroxine, so your metabolism slows up. Weight gain is one effect of this.

Treatment See your GP. He will take a blood test if he thinks you may have an underactive thyroid. It's easily treated with tablets, which you'll have to take for the rest of your life.

Other medical illness There are a few rarities which can cause weight gain, such as hormone problems and heart and kidney failure.

Treatment The chances that any of these problems will reveal themselves by making you put on weight are virtually zilch, as no doubt your GP will tell you if you see him. If he's unsure, of course, he'll run some tests.

Weight loss

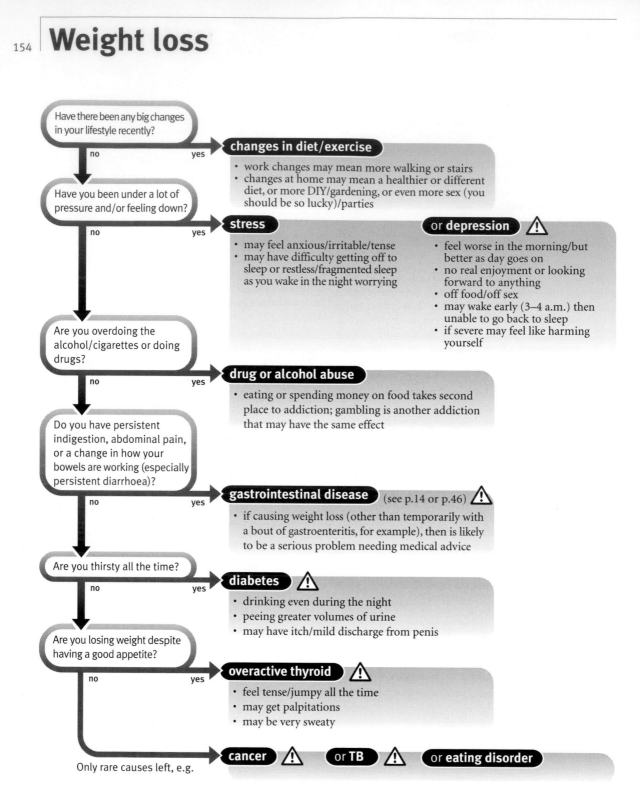

Have there been any big changes in your lifestyle recently?

no — yes →

changes in diet/exercise
- work changes may mean more walking or stairs
- changes at home may mean a healthier or different diet, or more DIY/gardening, or even more sex (you should be so lucky)/parties

Have you been under a lot of pressure and/or feeling down?

no — yes →

stress
- may feel anxious/irritable/tense
- may have difficulty getting off to sleep or restless/fragmented sleep as you wake in the night worrying

or depression
- feel worse in the morning/but better as day goes on
- no real enjoyment or looking forward to anything
- off food/off sex
- may wake early (3–4 a.m.) then unable to go back to sleep
- if severe may feel like harming yourself

Are you overdoing the alcohol/cigarettes or doing drugs?

no — yes →

drug or alcohol abuse
- eating or spending money on food takes second place to addiction; gambling is another addiction that may have the same effect

Do you have persistent indigestion, abdominal pain, or a change in how your bowels are working (especially persistent diarrhoea)?

no — yes →

gastrointestinal disease (see p.14 or p.46)
- if causing weight loss (other than temporarily with a bout of gastroenteritis, for example), then is likely to be a serious problem needing medical advice

Are you thirsty all the time?

no — yes →

diabetes
- drinking even during the night
- peeing greater volumes of urine
- may have itch/mild discharge from penis

Are you losing weight despite having a good appetite?

no — yes →

overactive thyroid
- feel tense/jumpy all the time
- may get palpitations
- may be very sweaty

Only rare causes left, e.g.

cancer   **or TB**   **or eating disorder**

⚠ If you have started to lose weight and feel very thirsty, you may be developing diabetes, and need to seek medical advice quickly.

Changes in diet/exercise There is normally a balance between the fuel you put in your body (in other words, what you eat) and the fuel you burn off (how much exercise you do). If this balance is shifted, the result will be a change in weight – so you'll tend to slim down if you exercise more or eat less.

Treatment Changes in weight of this sort are obviously normal – and good for your health if you were lardy to begin with.

Stress Being uptight all the time is another way of burning up energy; tension also tends to take away the appetite. The result: weight loss.

Treatment This is covered elsewhere – particularly in the 'Anxiety state' part of the 'Feeling tense' section (p. 59) and the 'Anxiety' part of the 'Palpitations' section (p. 103).

Depression Feeling very down often affects the appetite. Feeling tense may be a part of depression, too, and this will aggravate your weight loss. Depression is explained in more detail, and its treatment outlined, in the 'Feeling down' section (p. 57).

Drug or alcohol abuse Overdoing the booze or illicit substances can make you shed weight in a number of ways. It leads to a chaotic lifestyle, with eating properly being low on your list of priorities; it can cause anxiety and depression; it can bugger up your finances so you can't afford proper meals; it can cause illnesses (like hepatitis); and some drugs (such as amphetamines) simply burn off the calories.

Treatment Cut down – or better still, stop – the substance abuse and get a grip on your lifestyle. If you find it difficult and want help, check out your local drug or alcohol services (try the Citizens' Advice Bureau or the phone directory) or see your GP.

Gastrointestinal disease Your gastrointestinal tract starts at your mouth and ends at your back passage. Problems anywhere in between can make you lose weight. Examples include duodenal ulcer (which stops you eating properly – see the 'Gastritis/ulcer' part of the 'Abdominal pain – recurrent' section, p. 15) and inflammatory bowel disease or malabsorption (in which your food passes out as diarrhoea and so doesn't get absorbed into your system – see the 'Diarrhoea' section, p. 47).

Treatment If you have a gut problem severe enough to make you lose weight, you need to see your GP.

Diabetes This is explained, and the treatment described, in the 'Impotence' section (p. 69).

Overactive thyroid Weight loss is one of the many symptoms an overactive thyroid causes. For further details and advice about treatment, see the 'Excess sweating' section (p. 55).

Eating disorder This is the modern medical term for the different types of eating problems which used to be called anorexia or bulimia nervosa. They are much more common in women but do sometimes happen in men. People with this type of illness obviously have some psychological problem, but no one is quite sure exactly what brings it on.

Treatment Ideally, you should start to eat properly, stop any dieting tricks (such as using laxatives and making yourself vomit), and aim to get back as near to your 'ideal' weight as you possibly can. This is easier said than done – particularly as you may not agree that you have a problem. Friends and family are likely to try to persuade you to see your doctor. It's worth doing this, especially if you've lost a lot of weight, because eating disorders can sometimes make you really ill. Your GP may be able to help you with some simple advice and sort out any depression or anxiety which might be part of the problem. If he's not getting anywhere, or your illness is severe, he'll refer you to someone who specializes in this type of illness, like a psychologist or a psychiatrist.

Medical rarities Some small print medical conditions, such as cancer, TB, and AIDS, can cause dramatic weight loss, although there are usually lots of other symptoms which make it quite obvious that you're seriously ill.

Treatment If you think you might have one of these problems, see your GP asap.

Part Three

Live fast and die old

Are you confused about healthy living? Can't decide whether to keep fit and aim to live to 100 or to live for the moment and let the future take care of itself? Want to know how to enjoy life but still die old? Read on.

Life is for living and, for blokes, taking risks is part of it, as is having a good time. Who wants to spend a lifetime missing out on some pleasurable activity on the off chance that it will lengthen life span by a few months at age 80? By then, everyone you know will probably be dead and there will be no one left to party with. No one lives forever. If you manage to avoid dying of something age 79, then you can bet you'll die of something else soon after. That said, would you want to wake up dead one morning in your 50s (heart attack danger time) or even your 60s? Don't you deserve that pension you've paid so much into? Don't you want the opportunity to make a prat of yourself dancing at your kid's wedding?

So how do you get the balance right? How can you assess all the media hype about sensational breakthroughs; the conflicting advice of experts; and the sudden complete changes in medical opinion, all of which happen often enough to make you wonder if anyone really knows what they're talking about? For example, how would you feel if for years you'd been eating loads of fruit and veg – and spending a fortune on toilet paper – thinking you were helping to prevent cancer of the bowel, only to be suddenly told that doctors no longer believe that a high-fibre diet has any effect on this? Gutted. Yet that happened recently and it would be no surprise if the view changed back again in the future.

So giving advice can be tricky, but that's not going to stop us giving you some! Please note where we are coming from:

- We are not experts but we do deal with blokes every day and keep up to date with medical advances. However, others may disagree with our views and our interpretation of some medical research.

- We don't believe in eternal life but would like to live to at least 74, the average life expectancy for a man, enjoying life along the way.

- We don't mind whether you follow our advice or not, although we'd like you to be around to buy future editions of this book.

- We are natural sceptics and don't believe in doing anything that is going to be a lot of hassle for little pay-off.

- We shall only recommend changes that we reckon are worthwhile:
  ***** follow the advice if you possibly can
  *** follow the advice if it's not too much trouble
  * follow the advice if you like the idea

- Risk factors are factors which increase your chances of getting a disease in the future. However, there are no certainties! You can have all the risks and not get the disease or can have no risks and still get it. Life just isn't fair sometimes.

- If you're a lard-arse who only takes a fag out of his mouth to guzzle beer down it, then you may not be surprised to hear you have multiple risk factors for heart disease. These more than just simply add up (2+2+2 does not equal 6 but 8 or 9 or even 10), so even removing one of them can really make a big difference.

- The longer you have indulged in a risky behaviour the less likely its effects will be completely reversed by stopping. But that doesn't mean it's too late to stop – you can usually at least prevent more damage.

So much for the waffle. Now for some facts. Here is your blueprint for healthy living – the Bloke's Health Charter. Let's look at the do's and don'ts in more detail.

1. ***** **Get and stay hitched**. Great news: women are good for men. Having someone around much of the time at home will help relax you and improve your chances of being properly looked after. Compared to a married man, a never married man lives four years less. On the other hand, a divorced man also lives three years less than a married man, so it's worth waiting to make sure you have found the right woman.

One quirky fact is that married men unlucky enough to get a melanoma (skin cancer – nasty variety) are more likely to have it diagnosed early. Why? Because their partner spots it ands hauls them off to the doc.

2. *** **Do get laid at least twice a week** (***** if you can't then a DIY job will do just as well). The more orgasms you have the better, as sexual activity seems to have a protective effect on men's health – assuming of course that, if necessary, you have safe sex and make sure you don't catch anything nasty.

While shagging may be most fun, it's orgasms you're after, so if you have no partner to oblige then getting off by yourself is fine. Forget old jokes/old wives' tales: masturbating is not associated with any known bad effects (no, it doesn't cause stuttering or blindness). A quirky fact about shagging as opposed to masturbating is that couples who have sex at least three times a week look more than ten years younger than the average adult. We'd have thought they'd have just looked 'shagged out', but apparently not. Please note this youthful effect is only produced by regular sex in a good, strong, loving relationship and is not produced by shagging everyone in sight.

3. **** **Do have a good drink or two regularly** ***** BUT don't binge on the booze. More great news: a regular pint or two, or two or three glasses of wine on five or six days of the week probably does you good by providing some protection against heart disease and cancer.

All booze probably has much the same effect, though red wine is particularly rich in antioxidants which help prevent the damage to the body cells that causes serious illness. If you are really drinking for health then a glass or two a day of a recently produced Chilean Cabernet Sauvignon is best (smaller grapes allowed to ripen fully, as in Chile or Australia, give the highest antioxidant levels in the wine).

The government report Sensible Drinking reckons that up to about four units a day (1 unit = half a pint of ordinary strength beer or lager/a small glass of wine/a pub measure of spirits) is fine, but that if you regularly drink more than that then you may start to run into trouble. So four units a day or 28 units a week is not a target but a limit.

Unlike with sex, drinking more is not better but much worse! Regular heavy drinking (more than 50 units a week) will seriously damage your health, and going on a binge (11 units or more in one session) or getting too pissed too often is bad news too. When legless, you are a danger to yourself and others and run the risk of killing yourself drink driving, drowning, falling, or in fires (especially if you are a legless smoker), or even by suicide (remember booze doesn't necessarily make you happy). Then there's the hangover, which can boost cancer and heart attack risks as a side-effect of the nasty chemicals excess booze produces.

4. ***** *Do get fitter and leaner.* If you're a lump of lard then you're more likely to suffer from heart disease, high blood pressure, and diabetes. Your excess weight will be caused by a combination of overeating and, probably more importantly, underexercising (no, it is not caused by your glands – see the 'Weight gain' flow chart, p. 152). Sort out your eating habits by dieting (even losing 10 lb/5 kg or so over two or three months, no matter how fat you are, will make a significant difference) and stop being a slob by getting fit.

Getting fit or fitter is good for everyone whatever their weight. Seventy per cent of blokes don't take enough exercise – yet exercise reduces anxiety and depression and the risk of heart disease, and may help preserve new brain cells, so you get to keep your marbles in old age. If you go to a gym or health club for your exercise, it might also help you meet the love of your life and increase your chances of getting hitched or laid.

So, how much exercise is 'enough'? Vigorous activity – enough to get a bit out of puff – three times a week for 20 minutes each time is good (no, sex does not count as the puffing is from excitement, not exercise, and intercourse itself only lasts on average three minutes – not twenty!). Less vigorous exercise, like brisk walking, has an effect if done often enough (about seven hours per week).

Any fitness programme should start slow and build up gradually. Anabolic steroids are not about fitness but about the body beautiful, and are a big no no healthwise. Steer well clear of them.

5. *** *Do eat a healthy diet* (* *or at least take tomato sauce with everything*). But what is a healthy diet? A difficult question as there is loads of information and speculation about foods and what diseases they might or might not cause depending, for example, on how they're cooked and how much of them are eaten. Opinions and fashions change according to the latest research, which expert you listen to, and who's trying to sell their latest diet book. It boils down to this: as long as you are eating a fair amount of fruit and vegetables you are likely to be eating a healthy diet. You need balance in your diet and the rough proportions food groups should be mixed in are:

5–11 measures daily: bread, cereals, rice, pasta, potatoes

5–9 measures daily: fruit and vegetables (fresh, frozen, or canned)

2–3 measures daily: milk, yoghurt, cheese

2–3 measures daily: red meat, poultry, fish, Quorn, dried beans, nuts

Eat sparingly: fatty foods, sweets, sugary drinks, cakes, and confectionery. But the odd fry-up or Mars bar won't kill you, especially if you eat sensibly the rest of the time.

For your interest here are some (probable) food facts:

- Garlic has no effect on heart disease.
- Nuts contain fats that protect your heart.
- Chocolate – like red wine – contains heart-protecting antioxidants.
- Eating raw vegetables or salad three to four times a week reduces the risk of heart disease and cancer.
- Fats are necessary not only for their own sake but because they help us absorb vitamins A, E, and D.
- Ninety per cent of cholesterol is made by your body – so you can't lower your cholesterol level much by changing your diet.
- Cooked and processed tomatoes contain lots of antioxidants and have a beneficial effect on heart disease and cancer (tomato sauce with everything could reduce your risk of prostate cancer by 30–50%).

6. *** *Do get a life* * *BUT don't do Xmas shopping.* One in seven blokes will experience mental health problems and seven out of eight suicides each year are men. So 'having a life' and avoiding too much stress are both important parts of a healthy life. But advice on how to achieve them is far easier to give than to take.

However, the medical profession can sometimes cause stress by giving you advice which is more likely to create anxiety than actually prevent illness. For example, melanomas and skin cancers can be caused by too much sun exposure, but you don't need to avoid all sun as you would if you followed some of the current health advice. We don't believe it's worth getting too twitched about always keeping out the sun/using sunscreen/covering up, and so on to try and prevent skin cancer, but it is well worth taking care not to get sunburnt, especially if you are fair skinned. For example, sleeping off your hangover all day on the beach and burning the skin off your back is certainly not good for you. At the very least, it will ruin the rest of your holiday. Ideally you should keep out of the sun between 11 a.m. and 2 p.m. and sunbathe in short bursts.

Another example is cancer of the testicle where you might think you were really living dangerously by not examining yourself all the time. Yet only 1400 men a year in the UK are diagnosed as suffering from this, and 90% of them will recover. So, unless you are someone who feels better checking themselves regularly for lumps and doesn't get too anxious about it, we don' t really recommend it. However, that's not the same as saying that if you think there's something wrong with one of your balls you ignore it. If you notice a change, get to the doc pronto and get it checked out. Nor is it the same as saying that if your partner wants to check your balls for you (you should be so lucky) that you should be so impolite as to refuse.

And now here are some ways to keep mentally active:

- Make friends, as loneliness and isolation are bad news.
- Keep in contact with your parents.
- Keep interested in life; keep learning.
- Believe you're healthy; hypochondriacs are likely to die younger.
- Become a pet owner – a dog especially reduces stress, loneliness, and keeps you fitter.
- Get working – unemployment is bad for your health.
- Get rich – the more money you have the longer you will live.
- Support a good team (football or otherwise), especially one that wins regularly (all right, we know real fans can't help who they support and winning, unfortunately, has nothing to do with it) as the testosterone boost you get from victory is good for you.
- Don't go Xmas shopping as it will put up your stress levels and blood pressure and plays havoc with your bank account – except, of course, for shopping for a present for your wife/lover.

7. ***** *Don't smoke.* You may be bored with hearing this message but there is no doubt smoking is the greatest self-inflicted health risk of the lot. A smoker will knock, on average, six years off his life with massive extra risks of cancer and heart and lung disease, yet one in four blokes still smoke. Still, you have to admire them. They voluntarily pay an extra £20–30 a week in tax, knowing they are likely to kill themselves before they get their pensions, so saving the government a fortune. Everyone benefits except of course the smokers themselves and their families.

The good news is that giving up fags is likely, in time, to reduce your risks to nearly those of a non-smoker. For example, the risk of serious blood clots improves within two to three weeks of giving up and the risk of cancer of the lung is halved in five years. The risk from passive smoking to all those near and dear to you also drops. But remember – this applies to giving up, not cutting down, and not just changing to lower tar cigarettes. These are not much safer because you puff them more often and inhale more and deeper, so getting cancer lower in the lung.

If you normally grab your first fag of the day less than 30 minutes after waking up, then you are physically addicted to nicotine and your best chance of stopping is to use something like nicotine patches. For further details, see the 'Smoker's cough' part of the 'Cough' section.

8. ***** *Don't do drugs.* No one would recommend that anyone takes illegal drugs, nor has anyone ever shown that illegal drugs are in any way good for you. That said, government research shows that 45% of under-30s have taken an illegal drug at some point (15% in a given month), and that 10% have tried LSD, cocaine, or Ecstasy.

So if, despite advice to the contrary, you're determined to expand your mind the illegal way, you should choose and use your drugs carefully. According to the World Health Organization, cannabis is less addictive than alcohol or tobacco, and taking the odd spliff is hardly going to kill you, although it may land you in trouble with the law. But other drugs are far less predictable in their effects and far more likely to damage you. For example, cocaine or crack use can cause heart attacks, and anyone who gets onto heroin has a 50/50 chance of being dead within ten years.

If you think you have, or are developing, a drug problem and you can't stop yourself – get help – contact the local drug and alcohol advisory unit or your GP.

Key: ***** Follow the advice if you possibly can   *** Follow the advice if it's not too much trouble   * Follow the advice if you like the idea

Index